My Travels Through the Topic of Cancer

– PETER BERRY –

An environmentally friendly book printed and bound in England by
www.printondemand-worldwide.com

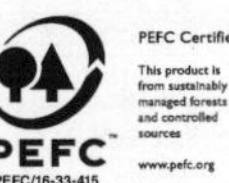

This book is made entirely of chain-of-custody materials

Published by books-on-line.net

On behalf of Peter Berry

My Travels Through the Topic of Cancer

ISBN: 978-1-909351-00-4

First published August 2012
Printed by
Printondemand-Worldwide
Peterborough, England.

Acknowledgements

Peter's book would not have been published without the fantastic support of UnLtd who encouraged Peter while he was writing it and later helped with the printing of this first edition.

The cover picture of *Cascade* was provided by James Beaton of Cascade Sailing, from whom Peter and Alan often hired the craft.

Foreword

I first met Peter Berry when we both worked for Barclays Life Insurance Company, in Barclays Bank in North Street Brighton. Both sharing an almost identical sense of humour, we quickly became close friends and kept each other in stitches for much of the time. Several people said to us, "I pity your poor wives!" which made us laugh even more.

It was impossible not to like Peter, for he was charming, would do his utmost to help others, with no care for himself and his needs. Although not the year, he shared September the 10th as his birthday with my beautiful wife, Jennifer, who was herself diagnosed with ovarian cancer a matter of months after Peter's passing. A double loss to a world where there is a distinct lack of kindly people.

I always hoped we would work together again, once I'd launched my organisation, then one day Peter called me, saying, "David! I have good news and bad news. The good news is I can at last come and work with you unpaid. The bad news is I have just been diagnosed with terminal cancer!" So he came with me to shows where we exhibited as, to use Peter's own words, my Stand Dolly. No one could have asked for a better friend.

At the end of the EIBTM in Geneva, we would have an extra night or two, which gave Peter the opportunity to take a boat trip on Lac Leman. I miss Peter and will never forget all the happy times we shared. I found reading Peter's book, as I checked the text, very uplifting, as I am sure will those who take the time to read this book.

David Aherne November 2010.

Peter Berry

Chapter One.

The early years.

The second world war was in its final throws when I was born in a private nursing home in Hillmorton Road, Rugby, Warwickshire, in September 1944. My mother, Sarah said that I was a small baby and that she could hold my bottom in the palm of one hand. “His little bottom was like two ripe plums”, she would relate to all and sundry whether they were interested or not, probably not, for other people’s children don’t have the same appeal as your own, do they?

My background has firm roots in the blue collar workers brigade, although it would be more accurate to describe it as being of the black collar genre. There was always a high degree of grime connected with the ‘heavy goods’ manufacturing industry of which my father, Horace was part. He was a ‘tin smith’, a sheet metal worker for BTH (British Thompson Houston) a major industrial conglomerate in Rugby, a company for whom his father worked in the transformer work shop. He was in what was described as in an ‘essential occupation’ and therefore did not see active service during the war, instead he was one of the ‘Dad’s Army’ brigade, a member of the Home Guard. I was never told of any heroics or jolly japes that went on, perhaps there weren’t any in those depressed and suppressed days of war-time. The one and only time my father had to come home from work before his shift was over, was when mother phoned the factory to say that I had gone missing. I was about four at the time and had set off on my own to the Fish and Chip shop, or 'tish shop' as I put it. A kindly neighbour found me in the next road and knew I shouldn't be wandering about on my own and took me home to a very relieved mother. Father wasn't too pleased as he'd lost half a day's pay but was happy I'd turned up safe and well. I can remember exactly what I was wearing all those years ago, black shorts, a hand knitted slipover in fawn with red trains running around the bottom, black Wellingtons and carrying a tin pop gun. I can't remember what I wore yesterday, but I do remember what I wore then!

Prior to their wedding, my mother who lived in Braunston, Northamptonshire, was in the service of a wealthy family who were, and still are, a household name in babycare products. It was not a normal event for women of a working class background to have their offspring in a private nursing home, but apparently nothing was too good for me. As The National Health Service had yet to be created, it was either a private nursing home or the state hospital where my sister, Pauline was born a few years before I came into the world as an afterthought, mother chose the former. Pauline is alleged to have said, "The whole world revolves around Peter," presumably that meant that meal times and other household duties were disrupted as our mother was too busy attending to my needs, of which no doubt there were many, as there still are! Mother had a surplus supply of Cash's name tapes left over from Pauline's school days, with P. J. Berry on them, so in the interests of economy, (particularly as the war was still on) I was christened Peter John to use the tapes up. I don't remember ever scrapping with my sister as we each had our own circle of friends in our respective age groups, although she still to this day reminds me that it was I who gave her chickenpox, I don't think she will ever let me forget it! By the time I had got used to the idea of having a sister, she went off to teacher's training college in

Norfolk, I saw very little of her except for the term breaks when she came home for six weeks or so at a time. When it was time for her to return, we would all bundle into our 1936 Morris 8 with a roof and boot rack piled high with trunks and suitcases. Cars didn't have heaters then, or our car didn't at any rate. If Pauline returned to college during the winter, Father would put a small paraffin stove in the car overnight and leave a sump heater, (also fuelled by highly combustible paraffin), under the car in the garage. Being wooden, the garage would have gone up like a torch if petrol had dripped from the carburettor onto the sump heater. Ordinary cars like ours did have leather seats, however and the distinctive smell is still embedded in my mind today. I sometimes accompanied mother on shopping trips to the nearby parade on Lower Hillmorton Road, the Co-op sold broken biscuits displayed in glass fronted tins which you were allowed to sample before buying, and Mother always asked the butcher for meat from a black cow. When queried, Mother would state, "It's all right, I always burn the meat and he thinks it comes from a black cow!" And I still choose the broken biscuits from a tin when offered instead of whole ones and prefer char-grilled steaks, old habits die hard. We used to be supplied with freshly killed rabbits, I don't know where from but I do remember taking the skins out to the Rag and Bone man who used to come down the road on his horse and cart ringing his hand bell and shouting an almost incomprehensible "Rag a Bone!" in a melodic tone. I would get to keep the threepenny bit, one new pence in today's money. Another 'tradesman' calling at the house would bring sausages and packets of leaf tea. I can recall to this day the bright orange paper packages of 1lb 'Orange Peeko Tips' which were stored in a dark stained wooden gramophone cabinet in the front room. The smell had permeated into the wood and was unforgettably pungent. The only thing that was curious about this delivery was that the goods arrived in a large dark blue van with chromium plated letters along the sides stating 'Lodge Plugs'. My godmother who lived opposite worked at the factory so no doubt it was part of the 'Old Boy' network.

My mother was an ambitious person, not only for wishing to improve the standard of living for herself and our father, but for us children too. The years spent in the service of others, made her realise the benefit and importance of acquiring material objects, such as owning your own home. The trend in those days, was to rent accommodation, which most people did, as before, during and immediately after the war as there was comparatively little job security. They bought a brand new house around the time my sister was born, much to the dismay of my father's family who thought that it would be a millstone round their necks for the rest of their lives and that my mother was being too pushy and trying to rise above her station. They paid approximately £350 for a semi-detached, three bedroomed house with a decent size garden in Richmond Road, Rugby, Warwickshire. According to my father the garden of their new house was full of builders' rubbish and debris. He had a theory that as it was the last one in the row to be occupied, all the people from the top end of the road would throw all the rubble they unearthed whilst digging and cultivating their garden, over their neighbour's fence. So by the time my parents moved in they had accumulated everybody else's rubble. There was a pair of houses subsequently built adjacent to us at N° 8, presumably they used the rubble that Father had thrown over the fence to make the foundations! Very few people had cars, so a garage wasn't included in the sale price of the house, ours was built some time after with allsorts of scrap wood father had accumulated. Whilst still learning to drive, he was a little heavy footed one day whilst parking the car in it and extended the garage by about three inches when all the nails pulled out of the bottom end wall! Double glazing had yet to be invented and central heating was considered unnecessary and would make people ill because there was no ventilation coming into the house. The sheer fact that there was ice on the inside of the windows during the winter months didn't seem to matter. Winter in those days ran from November to March and snow was almost certainly guaranteed at Christmas. Smog was a major factor in people's lives in those days and some people wore face masks to stop the 'pea soupers' getting onto their chests. Our milkman, 'Mac' could invariably be seen driving his electric milk float wearing a white mask and a pained expression on his face and one of those persistent coughs that comes to those with a propensity to pneumonia. On one occasion whilst our family was driving home from Coventry, past the Roots Group car factory at Ryton upon Dunsmore, the fog was so thick that the windscreen of our Morris 8, had to be wound open 90 degrees to facilitate a clearer view. It was a particularly cold journey back to Rugby about twenty miles away. It should only have been a twenty mile journey, but in fact took much longer. As we couldn't see more than a few feet in front of us, it seemed good sense (as my mother famously said at the time) to follow the removal van in front of us that had the name of 'Sam Robbins', a Rugby-based company. It was bound to be going back to its depot, or so she thought, in fact it was going on a removal job and took us miles out of the way towards Shipston-upon-Stour. We never tried that trick again! The smogs have gone, but the factory still remains, as a Peugeot car factory. Because our father earned comparatively good money as a skilled worker, there was always food on the table and reasonable quality clothes, some of which Mother used to make with her 'Jones' sewing machine, it was quite a momentous day when she bought an electric motor to fit on the side. My job of turning the handle on the machine to wind the bobbin was then defunct as I didn't have the co-ordination to slowly press the peddle, it was either 'flat out' or 'stop', I'm still like that now! I distinctly remember having a shirt made out of parachute silk, the seams of which were sewn in brown thread. Our shoes were made of leather, and our feet x-rayed to ensure the shoes fitted perfectly.

I was fascinated by the image in the x-ray machine, I could see my feet and all the dozens of tiny tacks and nails that went into making my shoes. There didn't seem to be the same concerns about exposing your children to the effects of the harmful x-rays in those days. The shoes were mainly bought from the Co-op so that a dividend, or "divi" would be payable. One of the first things I had drummed into me, after learning my name and address in case I got lost, was our dividend number, which is so indelibly printed onto my memory, it just trips off the tongue without a second thought, '12673'. So although my mother was a pre-Thatcherite in wanting home ownership, she didn't want to let collective consumerism fall by the wayside, which is probably a socialist trait that came out in her once a while.

There was never a more proud moment in my mother's life than in 1955 when their £300 mortgage had been repaid and they were sent the title deeds of the house. In those days the papers were very impressive with big seals and ribbons, not like today when all you seem to get is an N.H.B.C. certificate and a copy of the Land Registry certificate. I was shown the revered document whilst playing with my Hornby wind-up tin train on the lino flooring. I didn't really show much interest, well you wouldn't at that age, would you? I could make my engine spin round and crash into the skirting board, which was far more interesting than seeing it go round and round on its track, although the chips of paint on the floor always gave my game away and father something else to paint. It was the fashion then for kitchens and bathrooms (anywhere that there was steam) to be painted in a gloss finish. Our kitchen was painted cream and red, this combination was also the colour used by the London Midland Scottish (L.M.S.) railway company for its carriages in the 1950's. We schoolboys knew it as 'Blood and Custard' colour.

After completing her course at college in Keswick, Norfolk, my sister went on to become a teacher in Rugby, whilst I wasted my private education being more interested in handing out the pencils and being teacher's runner than studying. I had access to the school's stationery cupboard, it was an Aladdin's Cave of paper, rulers and pencils. I still can't resist stationers' shops and have enough ball point pens to last into the next millennium.

Father kept an allotment garden close to the local London & North East Railway station. During the golden age of steam, the shining leviathans in the blue livery colours of the L.N.E.R. would stop there on their way to and from Sheffield. The train of greatest grandeur that called at the station, carried the plaque of the "Master Cutler" reflecting the major industry of the city it was bound for. A boyhood game was to race the departing train up to the next road bridge about a quarter of a mile away. Although it was a close call, the train would always beat me to the bridge as my bicycle didn't have any gears, we couldn't afford them! I would have loved a bike with Derailleur gears, I would have even settled for a set of Sturmy Archers! The railway line has now been transformed into a cycle track and footpath. On the bridge was a small sweet shop, no bigger than a kiosk from where I bought misshapen sweet cigarettes and a glass of lemonade for six old pence.

I attended Eastlands School in Rugby for six years from 1949-1955, along with a number of neighbours' children and friends from other parts of the town. The school was next door to the Lodge Plugs spark plugs factory, who in the very early 1950's used huge steam powered Sentinel lorries with solid tyres and a whistle as loud as any of the railway engines on the adjacent L.N.E.R. track. When the whistle blew it would invariably send us all scampering away and there was many a bloody nose if you tripped over. Some of the pupils have been in touch with me after an absence of fifty years.

Following Eastlands, I went on to be educated privately at Longrood, an Edwardian school house at Old Bilton just outside Rugby, with Peter Carvell, the son of the bike and toy shop owner, from whom all my Christmas and birthday presents were bought. Naturally he had a bike with gears on it, which presumably was funded by my parents' patronage of his parents' shop, which is now an electrical equipment shop. I was envious of him at the time, as he had access to a whole stock room of toys, including the much-vaunted Hornby train sets. Although I had a Hornby wind-up train set made of tin, my treasured possession was a Trix-Twin electric train set. I still have it, all boxed up in the loft where it has been for the last, goodness knows how many years. At a recent model exhibition in Brighton there was a club stand for Trix-Twin owners, naturally, just like the visitors to the Antiques Roadshows, I wanted to have some idea of its current value. If I ever get desperate for a couple of hundred quid, I know how it can be raised.

My mother's family were canal folk. My grandfather, Isaac Merchant was captain and my grandmother Alice was helmswoman of a pair of seventy foot long Star-class narrow boats, *Arcturus* and *Sirius* which plied the canal network of Middle England operating out of the docks at Braunston.

During my mother's early years, she and her two sisters would accompany their parents on short runs, sleeping on board *Princess*, the butty boat. *Princess* would have been towed behind the motor-boat, *Prince*, and the girls helped with the locking procedure assisted by Peter, the black Pomeranian dog. A cine-film clip of my grandparents, their youngest daughter Ivy May who was tragically killed in a road accident before I was born, and showing Peter the dog, is currently being run on a continuous loop of film shown at the Waterways Museum in Gloucester Docks. It is some seventy years old and gives me a proud sense of belonging, seeing my family featured on film. The same film clip was shown on a recent re-run of Channel 4's 'Classic Ships' television programme.

Another film crew for Carlton television have recently shot footage for an inland waterways programme featuring Braunston Dock and Marina where my grandfather worked following his retirement from the boats. He made the rope fenders and his tools are still being used to this day at Braunston and it is believed that the film crew will include this in their documentary. My grandparents, Ivy, her sister Hilda whose son Michael died of Leukaemia aged just 22 years are all buried together in the cemetery at Braunston. It is widely understood, that I was named after the beloved dog, Peter, so in turn our daughter, Emma was named after her grandmother's dog, a scruffy little mongrel! Emma came from one of the houseboats converted from a wartime Motor Torpedo Boat, moored at Shoreham-by-Sea, where we now live. Later in the book there is an account of a man I met during my travels in France who converted the wooden built Motor Torpedo Boats into house boats just after the war. The dog my wife and I owned was a ruffian of a Wire Haired Fox Terrier called Shamus, so it will be interesting to see what my grandson will be called, if ever our daughter presents us with one! Shamus would have anything that moved, or would cock his leg over it if it didn't.

Because my background and upbringing was set in the industrial Midlands, my mother was determined that I should not follow in the footsteps of my father, and his father before him, by going into the manufacturing industry. She implored me to follow a career which didn't involve getting my hands dirty. She said that she had enough dirty clothes to contend with as it was. I never saw the bottom of the linen basket as it was always full. We were however, one of the few families who had a washing machine in the early 1950's. The factory my father worked in, made the metal casings for Hotpoint washing machines, and we had one of the prototype machines. The works parties at Christmas were always something to look forward to and if your father knew someone in another department of BTH, you would get to go to their party too.

We had a television set, which in 1950 was taller than me and had a screen about 9" square. In front of the screen hung a plastic magnifying screen to give at least 15" of viewing area, albeit everything had a distinctly blue tinge to it. This TV was like a little God sitting in the corner of the living room, it was polished just about every day and covered with a cloth at night like a sleeping bird. It was common during those early years of television, to have power cuts. We would sit and look at the blank screen by the light of a candle and hope that the interlude film of The Potter's Wheel, Swans or a Post Office information film would come bursting back to life in glorious monochrome at any moment. I recall seeing a news-reel announcing the birth of Brumus the Polar bear in London Zoo in 1950 and the Queen's coronation in 1953 with about twenty other residents of our road that were yet to have a television. During the transmission, if we had a power cut Mother made tea on the gas stove for us all and cut Eccles cakes into quarters to go round the assembled crowd. It was preferred by Mother, that I didn't engage in combative sporting activities either, this being due to my slight frame and petite stature. These attributes were however ideal for cross country running. There are few athletes who can lay claim to running along sections of the M1 motorway, which was being constructed in the mid fifties. The road ran within a mile of my school. Needless to say, running along earthworks can be quite a muddy pass-time and creates a great deal of washing. So I still got my hands dirty and just about everything else as well. My light frame and speed on the running track, earned me a place in the long jump final held during the school's sports day. I came second to a gangling six footer and walked away with prize money, equivalent today to around fifty pence. The private school was more like a holiday camp than a place of education. We had a swimming pool, which doesn't sound very grand today, but it was fifty years ago, albeit unheated. Luncheon was served by a chef wearing a traditional tall, white chef's hat and we had a roast joint every day that he would carve in front of us, plus trays of bread and dripping at break time and at the bell on Saturday morning. None of the other children in my road attended school on Saturdays, so I missed out on Saturday morning matinees at the local cinema. Cholesterol wasn't heard of in those days, in fact the reverse was stated, "a good layer of fat would line your tummy and keep out the cold!" How things have changed. Sadly the school is no longer in existence and houses now occupy the site. I used to catch the bus to school, it was operated by the Midland Red Bus Company, whose slogan was "The Friendly Midland Red". However one particular conductress would let us on the bus and then bawl out, "Sit down, keep your feet in and shut up!" Very friendly.

Family holidays were taken every year at the seaside. We were fortunate to be able to take them, as not every family could afford to do so. In the main, we stayed at guest houses and the nearest seaside resort to Rugby was Skegness in Lincolnshire, or 'Skeggy' as it was affectionately known. Rhyll in North Wales was also a popular destination for people living in the Midlands. Going in the opposite direction, Bournemouth and Great Yarmouth were resorts visited by our family during the 1950's. One year we spent a holiday at Gorlestone near Great Yarmouth accompanied by a friend of my sister's. I couldn't do any running around like most other 9-year-olds as my leg was swathed in bandages following a scalding accident at home a week before we departed. My mother had been doing the weekly wash and her hands were still soapy which caused the tea pot to slip out of her hand. The scalding hot tea went down my leg and hurt like blazes. As I tried to pull down my thick woollen sock, the skin came away with like a second sock revealing a red raw area of flesh. I had to be rushed to hospital and penicillin soaked square bandages were applied to my leg and yards of bandage. I received a great deal of attention on that holiday but it's no substitute for being able to run around and play in the sand. On one trip to Bournemouth, we arrived too late to find board and lodgings, so we bunked down in the car overnight. There were bright red lights shining into the car all night and in the cold grey light of dawn we saw that we had parked on the slip road of the chain link ferry from Poole to Sandbanks. Mother went mad as she couldn't swim. We booked into a B&B the next night at 10/6 (.52p in today's money). I didn't think that money was that tight for my parents but it obviously was. I can remember constantly asking for ice creams sold from those seafront tricycles with cool boxes on the front and a man in a white coat and a straw hat. I was given two old pence to buy just the wafers and no ice cream. When our daughter was small and constantly asking for treats, I would relate this tale and usually it worked.

On a holiday to Portsmouth in 1952, I vividly remember scrap yards piled high with crashed aeroplanes, some British, but mainly German machines. What would aircraft restorers give to stumble upon such a wealth of WWII history today? By the pier, adjacent to the railway station at Portsmouth Harbour, were small boys who would retrieve pennies from the seething mud. They were collectively known as 'Mud Larks' and there was no shortage of people prepared to throw coins to them, just to see them scrabbling about getting absolutely filthy. You could almost imagine the look of dismay on my mother's face, she would have loved to have given them a good scrub down and send them home clean and tidy. She had an obsession with cleanliness and would wash everything in sight. She once said that she would like to scrub the Plaza steps in Rugby, it was a grand picture house and had marble steps that ran up to the main entrance. She would not have allowed anyone to walk on the gleaming marble afterwards, but her pleasure would have been in seeing the steps shine and sparkle.

Her eagerness to clean everything in sight didn't always extend to laundry however, as the following passage explains. One Sunday morning, during the summer months, I announced to my parents, who were sitting, reading The Sunday Express, that I was to marry Angela Franklin, my girlfriend when we were both about seven or eight. Angela lived half way up the road on the same side as us and is younger than me by a couple of months. We would play street games with the other kids in the road, there were probably only about ten of us in the whole road which consisted of about one hundred houses and practically no cars to bother us or obstruct our games. Mother said I couldn't get married as it was the weekend and I didn't have a clean shirt, and she certainly wasn't about to wash and iron one for me! Life can be very cruel when you're seven or eight and not capable of doing your own laundry.

I am still in touch with Angela and her husband today some fifty years on from my proposal. Quite by chance, my wife, Julie and self were travelling on the French Railway's TGV from Geneva to Paris and were sitting next to a couple who we established were from Rugby. It transpires that not only were they living in the road in which I had been brought up, but Angela was looking after their house whilst they were away. It's a small world. We have subsequently met up and continue to do so. I wrote to The Rugby Advertiser stating that I was hoping to visit the area after an absence of forty-five years, and does anyone still remember me. The response was very encouraging and I met up with former school chums and received a letter from a lady for whom Angela had been bridesmaid, and who went to school with my sister.

Despite being a major industrial centre, Rugby was not extensively bombed during WWII, unlike Coventry 20 miles away, which was a popular haunt of my mother's for buying dress making materials. At an early age I was already familiar with Moygashell, Seersucker and Mercerised cotton. It was not surprising that when I left school, I should follow an occupation in the retail clothing industry. I had a head start on the range of fabrics available and the way in which they were woven, and it didn't involve getting my hands dirty either! When I came out of school on a Saturday, particularly if father had gone to football, I would go to the children's clothes shop that mother worked in, Overton's of Regent Street, Rugby and hang around the alteration workshop with all the alteration hands. We would have 'Camp' coffee and iced buns during the morning. Having left Rugby in 1957, our family settled in Surrey. Guildford was then a pleasant country town, but today it resembles a London suburb with shopping centres and chain stores. I joined a privately owned clothing store that had six branches between Guildford and London. I was the junior who polished the brass edges to the glass topped counters and was delegated to make the morning and afternoon tea. I had never made a cup of tea in my life but had observed from my mother, the process involved. I must have got it right as I kept that exalted position for six months before the next junior joined the company and took over my job. I worked in the High Street, at the bottom of which ran the River Wey. It had a small wharf and moored in it was the narrow boat, *Arcturus* which my grandparents used to operate. It was as if my mother's childhood past was following her. She disliked the connection between her working class background and the new life she had forged for her family. She did everything possible to erase the memory of the austere past, even to the point of denying that she was born on the butty boat *Princess*, which we believe to be the case. My grandfather, Ike as he was known, offered to give me a wooden narrow boat when I was about 17 yrs. Quite rightly my mother said, "And where do you think you're to put it?" Today, if you can find a classic wooden boat, it would cost a small fortune, I never did get to own a narrow boat. Seventy years after the boats, *Arcturus* and *Sirius* were sold and went their respective ways, they are together again and currently moored in Hertfordshire.

Through a chance encounter, my sister met the current owner of *Arcturus*, Bryan Nicoll. Michael, Bryan's son now owns *Sirius*. The Star-class boats built by Walkers of Rickmansworth in 1934 are numbered consecutively 28 & 29 and are a waterways legend. I occasionally get the chance to visit the boats at canal boat rallies. Guildford was a good town to live in during the 1960's, with a friend or two, we used to attend the dances at the recently opened Civic Hall. Bands such as Dave Berry and The Cruisers, Brian Poole and The Tremeloes and The Swinging Blue Jeans used to perform. We also saw Eric Clapton and The Yard Birds at The Plaza in Guildford, long before they reached international acclaim. Acker Bilk was also a regular on the pub circuit, together with The Temperance Seven with their syncopated rhythm, but they needed a large stage for their act and would appear live at the Odeon at the top of the High Street. London was only 30 miles away and we would regularly make trips up there, thinking ourselves to be very decadent, wearing thick, knitted cardigans and suede shoes long before the hippy movement adopted the style. If we went to "Town", the Surrey saying for London on a Sunday, a suit was invariably worn. As I worked in a store that made bespoke suits, I could have one made in what ever style and material I chose. Girls during that era were wearing twin-sets and pearls with flowing calf length skirts and bobby socks, straight out of the 1950's American movies like Sandy from Grease. Having an income for the first time in my life gave me the opportunity of owning all the latest electrical equipment such as; a reel to reel tape recorder, leather cased transistor radio, a boat and a car! I had private driving lessons that cost 10/6 (.52p) per hour and was taught by an ex-policeman. He knew every police-woman in Guildford, for in those days the police still walked the streets before their numbers were reduced and Panda cars were introduced. Needless to say, most of my tuition was spent balancing the car on the clutch and accelerator up the numerous hilly side streets of the town whilst he chatted to the W.P.C.'s! An ex-boss once complimented me on my hill start abilities whilst visiting clients in the hilly side streets of Brighton. Guildford's hilly streets leading down to the river did have their drawback however. During one winter, when a higher than average rain fall was encountered in the town, I saw the grand pianos from the music store immediately adjacent to the river, floating in the basin at the foot of the High Street. Fifty yards away from the bus station and the wharf where *Arcturus* was moored. The entrance to Alby John's dance school was there too and by another coincidence of life, it is where the wife of a fellow patient at the hospital in Worthing, which I attend and has the same medical condition as myself, also learned to dance, as she too lived in Guildford. She also was part of the circle of acquaintances who attended various parties and a memorable barbecue on the water-meadows adjacent to the river. The event was memorable for not remembering how I got home, or how my friend got back to his lodgings either, which was a little worrying as he was driving! I have seen both of the aforementioned people, forty years after leaving Guildford. It really is a small world! One of the most embarrassing moments as a junior of the store in town where I worked, was when an adjacent departmental store closed its doors and our window dresser bought some of the female mannequins. It was I to whom the task of carrying them up the High Street to our own store was delegated, where do you put your hands on a naked female model without drawing attention to yourself? Whilst working in Guildford, I had the chance to study at Queen's College, Cambridge, I was only there for a week and it was work related, still it sounds good, doesn't it? I was a member of the National Association of Outfitters and was up for a nomination to fly out to New York to see what influence the American clothes market would eventually have on our own domestic scene, sadly I didn't win, I would have loved to have flown in a Boeing 707. My parents moved from Guildford in 1963, technically I was still living "at home" and had been on a continental holiday to Jugoslavia. A friend and I who worked in Guildford, at the same company as the girl 'Flick' I mentioned earlier, went on a Cosmos holiday which cost nineteen Guineas, (£19.95p) we stayed in Opatija, which was the Austro-Hungarian equivalent to Monaco and had grand buildings and wide boulevards. The country was still under a communist regime at that time and Marshall Tito's bust was very much in evidence throughout the town, as were tanks and the militia. Whether or not my parents thought I should never be seen again for venturing into such a remote and hostile environment, I do not know. When I returned, they had moved house and someone else was living in the family home! Were they trying to tell me something do you suppose? A phone call to my sister in Horsham saw her collect me from Guildford and provided me with accommodation for the night before tracking down my parents the next day. They had moved into temporary accommodation whilst their new house was being completed, the new purchaser was anxious to move in, so my parents moved out. We all moved back to Guildford at a later date before finally all moving together in 1966 to Eastbourne. I was working at a clothes store in Brighton, some 30 miles distant. The daily travelling was proving too expensive as the car I was driving consumed as much oil as it did petrol. I was offered the chance to rent the spare room from our lady window dresser. She was a vegetarian and gave me a fried egg and tinned tomatoes every morning for breakfast.

During the time I worked in Brighton, I met my future wife, Julie. She worked at the company's Hove branch, opposite St Andrew's church where we married two years later in 1970. Some of the staff were able to lean out of the stock-room windows to see us emerge from the church. The husband of the lady who I regarded as an aunt, was in service with my mother some fifty years earlier, was a Special Policeman. He halted the Saturday morning traffic along Church Road in Hove whilst our entourage walked across the road to a nearby hotel where the reception was held. There were no luxury limos in those days to transport the guests, we walked in the bitterness of April winds, which did wonders for the girls' bouffant hairdos!

Our daughter, Emma, was born in December of the following year in a maternity hospital in Rustington, West Sussex. Legend has it that if an expectant mother saw the rabbits on the lawn of the hospital, she would return within two years to have her second child. We never did see the rabbits, so Emma is an only child. Most of our married life was spent in the seaside village of Rustington, over which the sound barrier was broken in 1953 by Neville Duke in a Hawker Hunter jet aircraft. I became a governor of a private girls' school, and served on the committees of the village hall and allotment society. These were all useful contacts for me whilst carrying on my profession as an estate agent in the village for a multi-national insurance company. Although the activity that brought me most notoriety, was being part of the amateur theatre troupe. On one memorable February morning, I was lighting my briar pipe from the burning embers of my bonfire, when I was approached by a fellow allotment holder. His head was bowed and turning from side to side whilst audibly tutting at me saying, "Who would have thought it, you of all people!" I asked why me of all people and why wouldn't anyone have thought it? The question came from someone who was obviously not at ease with the juxtaposition of painting grease on the axle of my rather squeaky wheelbarrow and the grease paint used in stage make up. He had seen the write up in the local paper of my performance on stage as Frank Gibbons, the father in Noel Coward's wonderful play, This Happy Breed. "How could you shovel manure around in the morning and parade about on stage wearing make up in the same evening?" I told him that the principle was just the same, you simply address the vegetables sitting in neat rows in front of you! Having the allotment garden invariably meant a glut of fruit and vegetables were produced, some were bartered for other produce amongst the other allotment holders and some were sold.

Next door to the office in which I worked, there was a green grocer who would take any surplus from me and sell upon my behalf. One day the proprietor came to me and asked, "Can we have some more of your Rhubarb? I don't know what the old ladies do with it, but they can't buy enough of it!" I assumed it was coming up to jam making time for the Women's Institute, I sold pounds and pounds of it, not only in weight but in monetary terms too. As I still had huge amounts of surplus fruit and vegetables, I decided to embark upon a project of making home made wine, and that's when the fun really began.

I would bring home peas in their shells for freezing, which meant blanching them before cooling and subsequent freezing. The boiling water used to blanch the peas would then be used for making into wine by adding yeast and sugar. This process killed two birds with one stone as a separate process to obtain the taste and colour from boiling the vegetables was no longer required. The economics of the process didn't stop there because the spent pea shucks were taken back down to the allotment and added to the compost heap which was subsequently dug into the ground for next year's vegetable production, it was the tail wagging the dog! I also made wine from soft fruits such as raspberries, a much longer and slower process than vegetables that remained whole during the steeping process. We had not long had a new kitchen fitted to our house which was my wife's pride and joy. The work tops were red and the cupboard doors and twin sink unit was pure white. I had been steeping the raspberries in a gallon bucket of water standing on the new work top and given my solemn promises not to make a mess. Now for anyone who has ever made wine from raw ingredients rather than a kit from Boots, you would know how shallow that promise was, it's absolutely impossible to make wine without making some form of mess, and boy, did I make a mess! Knowing that it was likely that a serious amount of ear-bending would be conducted if I attempted to strain the pulp of the raspberries whilst my wife was hovering around in the kitchen, I decided to wait until she had gone to bed. Things started off well enough, I rolled up the sleeves of my shirt and had a bowl of water at the ready to rinse myself off should it be necessary to do so. The raspberry pulp was tipped little by little into the conical shaped 'jelly bag' to strain off the pips so that just the juice went into the demijohn for subsequent fermenting. This process was however taking far too long for my liking, so I set about squeezing the jelly bag to assist the separation process. To the naked eye, the stitch holes in a jelly bag looked as if they were so small and would not allow liquid to come out of them even under pressure, however in reality these holes were nothing more than potential fountains which allowed copious amounts of brightly coloured fruit juice to spurtle everywhere. The work tops were covered in a fine mist of red juice as were the cupboard doors, my shirt and all the uncovered areas of skin. I got into an awful mess, but once rinsed off I was ready to repeat the process until the last drop of juice had been extracted from the pulp. Not wanting to make too much mess of my remaining clothing, I stripped down to my undershorts believing that it is easier to wash skin than it is a pile of clothing. Bright red pulp stained my hands, wrists and lower arms, it looked as if I had committed a massacre and cut up the victim's body for disposal. It was of course at this point that my wife entered the kitchen to be greeted by the sight of her near naked husband with blood red hands, and a particularly guilty look on his face. It was probably at this point that I decided to give up wine making, or it could have been three weeks later when the fruits of my labours were fermenting in a demijohn in the airing cupboard, and exploded. This caused considerable concern, not just because it chose to explode at 2 o'clock in the morning, but because the entire contents of the said airing cupboard were stained red. Sheets, shirts, pillow cases, underwear, you name it, it was dyed and even when washed vigorously managed to remain a delicate mulberry colour. That was the end of my venture into home made wine.

When our daughter Emma was living at home with us, we only ventured abroad for holidays on two occasions. We didn't want to put our dog, Shamus into boarding kennels, so we bought a touring caravan and spent most summers in Cornwall. We haven't been back since, favouring continental destinations with hotel accommodation that doesn't require you to put wellies on and trudge across a field to go to the toilet. In 1992, I was blamed single-handed for the decline in the property market, and was made redundant after almost twenty years with the company. I needed to secure another position quickly and rang round to all those companies that I understood what their core business activities were. I was intrigued by the manner in which job interviews had changed during the twenty years of monogamous employment. Interviewers weren't interested in my capabilities for the job applied for, they wanted to see if I could think outside the box. "Tell me if I should build a new headquarters out of town with acres of staff parking spaces, or refurbish this existing town centre office with no parking facilities," asked one prospective employer. Fortunately, being an ex-estate agent, I came up with a plausible answer. The truth be known, I quite enjoyed hawking myself around southern England in search of a new position. At one office, I entered and waited for someone to acknowledge my presence. When they didn't I said in my most assertive (and dramatic) voice, "I'm here on the instructions of Norman Tebbitt, I've been made redundant, I've got on my bike and wish to see the hirer and firer, now!" By the end of the week, I had three job offers and accepted a post within financial services, which was an industry with close links to estate agency, so I found it very easy to adapt to my new position. I studied for the industry's professional examinations and passed, which was some achievement as I had failed the finals of the estate agents' examinations on three occasions. I didn't expect to be studying for exams forty years after leaving school. Perhaps I should have paid more attention at school instead of being pencil monitor.

The insurance company that was my most recent employer, had its head office in Peterborough, Cambridgeshire. We came across the city by accident whilst en route to York for our final holiday in our touring caravan. Peterborough, being half way up the country, made an ideal stopping off point. The Caravan Club site was situated in a country park, around which were miles and miles of cycle paths, all completely away from traffic and most importantly, flat! We loved it there and would consider hiring a caravan with the sole purpose of utilising the cycle track facility, even though we may have to put our wellies on to go to the toilet.

Having been with the insurance company only a few months, I started complaining of severe back ache whilst driving up to their head office from Brighton during the winter in a bright yellow convertible Ford Escort. My colleagues called it a 'hairdresser's car'. My mother, who had an explanation for most things in life, had for years advocated that drivers of Ford cars always suffered from bad backs. She even coined the expression 'Ford Back' when symptoms of back pain were described to her. She was very astute when diagnosing medical conditions, but even she could not possibly have known what disease I was suffering from. As my condition was worsening rather than showing any signs of improvement, I sought medical advice, the eventual outcome changed my life completely.

Chapter Two.

The Bombshell.

No one likes to consider the possibility of contracting a serious illness, it's not a very pleasant thought, so when it happens, it's totally devastating. In my own mind, I had always regarded the contracting of cancer as a little like winning the Premium Bonds, it always happens to someone else, never to you. Imagine then someone telling you that this time it is you, and there's no jackpot prize to look forward to.

I suppose I had been very fortunate as a child, and kept remarkably well, apart from the 'run of the mill' childhood aliments such as chickenpox and measles. I had escaped all other serious conditions which were prevalent during my childhood, such as the outbreak of polio in Coventry just twenty miles from where I lived, which took a serious toll on young lives. Those who survived and were not put in an 'Iron Lung' for the rest of their short lives, were deformed by the illness, people such as the late Ian Drury of the Blockheads. During the early fifties, it was an illness that every mother was petrified of her offspring contracting. I was small, beautifully formed, but light framed, accordingly my mother would attempt to 'dose me up' with all kinds of preparations in order to make me grow or bulk up a little. I was given the most horrendous liquid medicine called 'Phosphorine' which was almost neat iron and made my teeth fur up as if I'd been chewing raw, under-ripe rhubarb, which on reflection would have probably been more palatable. What with this stuff and spoonfuls of 'Virol' malt and cod liver oil, my body was producing much more blood than I needed, which resulted in violent nose bleeds and trips to the doctor. I recall as quite a young child being taken to Dr Parker's surgery and slipping on an unsecured carpet runner. This rug propelled me several feet along the highly polished floor. I've always been a person to say what he thinks and is appropriate for the occasion, I said "I wish [sic] you wouldn't polish this floor so much!" Not the sort of thing that a four-year-old would be expected to say to a professional person. Mother was of course told that she was over feeding me with blood generating products and should discontinue the practice immediately, but mothers know best, don't they and I continued to suffer from nose bleeds until the time I got married and left home. I wasn't a regular visitor to the doctor and can't recall a time when I would have needed to take a day off work through illness. I did have to go and have a lump of rusting Volkswagen exhaust pipe removed from my eye as I had unwisely attempted to change the silencer myself and failed miserably. But for pure medical problems, I hardly ever went to the surgery. I did attend a pre-employment medical at the general practitioner's near to where I currently live, he gave me a clean bill of health and my prospective employers offered me a full time position with them. In the light of what has subsequently happened, if I were the employer, I would have filed a law suit against the doctor, for clearly I was not at all the well person he made me out me to be. During the first few weeks of my new employment for a Cambridgeshire based insurance company, I began to experience a degree of lower back pain. This I attributed to carrying a pilot's case around containing one each of all the forms my employer had ever printed, plus a laptop computer and printer. The total weight was around seventy pounds and it hurt my back considerably. During the training course which all new recruits had to attend, I had the opportunity of playing squash as the building in which we were based, was the company's sports centre. I thought that all the sitting around during the day was seizing my back up and a bit of exercise would do me the power of good. I had always been a keen squash player, so it was exercise to which I was accustomed. I only played one game, but was pleased to win it. I didn't go on to play badminton with the others and opted for snooker instead which I thought would be a little kinder to my back. However all the bending over the table to take a pot shot hurt like crazy and I retired injured.

When I had returned to my district and started to call upon clients, it reached the point where I would ask my immediate line manager to accompany me on my appointments just to carry my equipment, not good working practice as it was time consuming and not cost effective to the company. I decided to seek help from the medical profession and arranged to see my local general practitioner who it transpired was on holiday and I had to see another doctor in the practice, she turned out to be less than helpful, and made the comment that most people experience some degree or other of back pain and with rest it should go away. For some that may be so but for me it wasn't. After a week's rest, the pain was not getting any better. In fact it got worse as time went on. This was early April 1998 and the diary entries which chronicle my experiences, follow;

Thursday 16th April 1998

Pain no better, saw local G.P. in Shoreham-by-Sea. I was told that "It's muscle pain, go and see a physiotherapist!" I should have insisted on a blood sample being taken.

I returned to the surgery and was advised that a course of treatment with a local physiotherapist was recommended at no cost to me, it was all to be on the National Health Service. Appointments were made and I duly attended, albeit in a great deal of pain, meeting a former client there who was also having 'back problems' which is Britain's foremost ailment in terms of time taken off work. The only medication I was taking at that time was an Ibruprofen rub bought over the counter at Boots, which brought little or no relief. The bed in the surgery had to be lowered to the floor to allow me to get on it, this should have been an indication to the practitioner as to how much pain I was experiencing, but it wasn't as the tale reveals. Together we embarked upon four of the six weeks' treatments I was due to receive, I hadn't had acupuncture before and didn't quite know how it would feel, but my mind was put at rest that it would be a pleasurable experience and not at all painful, just a warm feeling bringing relief and would mask out any signs of pain, however! This use of acupuncture necessitated the insertion of ten, eight inch needles either side of my spinal column in the hopes that it would relieve the pain, it didn't and at one point I was asked to let go of the practitioner's leg. She took offence and didn't like being grabbed and mistaken for the upright support of her own table. It was not entirely my fault, she shouldn't have been standing so close, or hurt me so much!

Wednesday 22nd April 1998

Appointment with physiotherapist, pain getting worse not better. Didn't help when acupuncture needles were inserted into either side of my spine. Last treatment due on 06/05/1998 and I can't wait for it all to be over and done with.

I returned to the local doctor's surgery in even more agony than before. I found that I couldn't sleep at night from the acute pain no matter how I tried to position myself against the unpleasant feeling, walking was extremely difficult and only achieved by the use of a hiking pole which I'd brought back from a holiday in Austria and driving a car was completely out of the question. Something had to be done, and soon. I was referred to the local hospital, just ten minutes' walk away from the surgery, for a blood test, that surely must reveal if anything was not right. I could tell by the look on the phlebotomist's face that things were in fact, far from being right. She advised me that the hospital in

Worthing would contact me in due course, which turned out to be within two days, that's how concerned they were for my health and well being.

Wednesday 20th May 1998

Awaiting results of blood tests. I've got a premonition that I may soon be unable to travel. Took myself off to London by train and visited a travel poster exhibition at The Victoria & Albert museum. Saw also Canary Wharf and the Cutty Sark *at Greenwich. I seized any chance to get out and about, I may not be able to soon. After a reasonable night's sleep, dosed up to the eyeballs, I awoke and still felt reasonably well, but the pain was persistent and wouldn't go away, but I wasn't going to let it stop me. I had always had an interest in 1930's travel posters and decided to make the journey to London's Victoria and Albert museum, I felt well enough to travel and was determined to cram as many excursions into the next few weeks in case I became grounded later on, I'm glad I did. We had also arranged an 80th birthday outing for my wife's mother, we were off to the Isle of Wight. We met up with Julie's parents at Lancing in West Sussex and caught South Downs 700 bus service to Portsmouth Harbour, initially we sat on the top deck to get a good view. Although we travelled on a road which I had driven along on countless occasions, I only ever saw hedgerows and roofs, never into the front gardens of houses, so this was a good opportunity to do so.*

By the time we had reached the City of Chichester, (approximately 30 miles away) the jolting on the top deck became too much for my poor old back and the pain became excruciating, so we moved down stairs and I wedged myself against the front bulkhead, behind the luggage rack at the front of the bus. By doing this I was able to brace myself against jolts and the subsequent pain they brought. We eventually arrived at Portsmouth Harbour and caught the Wight Link fast catamaran boat service to Ryde on the Isle of Wight. You would have thought that the bouncing around on top of waves would be uncomfortable, but it wasn't as the fluid motion of the boat through the water brought no discomfort at all. We had an all inclusive ticket which granted travel on the island's railway to Shanklin. There used to be a steam railway in existence on the island, now steam trains are only to be seen at the working museum track at Haven Street. We, on the other hand used the ex-London Transport Underground electric trains which now ply the route to Shanklin on the other side of the Island. To say it was bumpy is an understatement, the track is far from straight, level or even, therefore the pain which I had described as excruciating on the bus, was now at the point of being indescribable! I had to 'strap hang' all the way as I couldn't sit down because of the jolting, it was also painful for me to reach above my head to reach the leather strap. I was in such pain I couldn't speak. It required every atom of my concentration just to remain as calm and collected as I could. It came as a pleasant relief to sit still and eat a light lunch, which I spun out to last as long as possible just to remain seated. The journey home was just as uncomfortable as the journey there, but at least I knew how to position myself to get optimum relief from all the jolts and bumps.

During that same week an appointment had been made for me to attend Worthing Hospital's haematology clinic to see the consultant, Dr Tony Roques. I was in a great deal of pain by now and not really able walk any distance, so for the convenience of all, I was transported in a hospital wheelchair up to the Pathology Dept. As soon I entered his office, he could tell by the way I was walking how much pain I was suffering and said he had a fair idea of the cause of my problem, but would need to conduct tests to confirm his suspicions. The test comprised the insertion of a hollow needle, an auger type of implement which he drilled into my hip bone, to tap into the soft bone marrow that lay within the bone. It sounds painful, and it was. The fluid he extracted was of similar to the viscosity of glycerine, and about the same colour. My wife was present throughout the consultation and felt for me as the auger was wound into my pain-wracked body. She could see both the tears welling in my eyes and determined look on my face that I would endure this procedure without the use of anaesthetics. When the procedure was conducted on other occasions I would insist on being 'knocked out', it's a strange sensation in that you are able to respond to instructions, but remember nothing of the procedure at all except for the nurses telling you that you swore at the consultant whilst under the anaesthetic, he still speaks to me though so it couldn't have been that derisive. We were advised that the biopsy report would take about a week, but the haematologist thought he could confidently predict that I was suffering from Multiple Myeloma, (Bone Marrow Cancer). It is a rare form of cancer and perhaps best described as a cross between Leukæmia and Osteoporosis. It affects the plasma cells found in white blood cells in the 'B' lymphocytes of the blood and reduces the body's own natural defence system, damages the kidneys and softens the bones making sufferers susceptible to bone fractures, more than a dozen people are diagnosed with the disease every day in Britain and the attrition rate is almost 2, 500 every year. There is no cure at present and its cause is not known, but exposure to chemicals and radiation is thought to trigger it. I blame the Russians for my condition and the Chernobyl nuclear power plant explosion which showered the whole of southern England with radioactive fall out. A report which follows, was from an article I submitted to Reuters for publication.

I BLAME THE RUSSIANS!

The Russian president, Vladimir Putin had been criticised by his fellow countrymen and the whole of the outside world, for the seemingly excessive use of chemicals during the siege to recapture the Moscow theatre from the Chechnyan rebels on 26th October 2002. The relatives of the victims were understandably up in arms over the indiscriminate use of the opiate chemical spray Trimethyl Fentanyl, or possibly the even more devastating BZ gas which the Americans no longer use as it is deemed to be too unpredictable and dangerous. Both agents were developed during the cold war and generally used on trained, fit soldiers out in the open air. Whichever gas was used, it was on mainly elderly theatre goers who hadn't eaten for three days and whose resistance to such a gas was diminished by those factors, so it had a devastating affect. The potential long term effects on the health of these victims isn't and cannot be known for many years to come. I too consider myself to be a victim of the long term effect of Russian toxins to which I was subjected following the explosion at the reactor in Chernobyl on 26th April 1986. Vast areas of the southern part of England where I live were generally accepted to be subjected to the poisonous gamma radiation clouds emitted after the explosion. Some eight years after the nuclear fallout. I was diagnosed with a form of cancer that affects the bone marrow for which there is no known cure at present. The information produced in leaflets supplied by the cancer organisations all claim that this form of the disease is caused by exposure to chemicals and pollutants. As I have never been exposed to these during my private or working life, it is my widely held belief that my form of cancer could only have been caused by exposure to the harmful toxins such as discharged from the Russian explosion. Whilst I was undergoing treatment in Hammersmith Hospital, London, my room overlooked the famous, or infamous Wormwood Scrubs prison, ironically the Russian word for Wormwood, is Chernobyl!

Friday 22nd May 1998

Attended appointment with specialist, Dr Roques in Worthing. He broke the news that I was suffering from Multiple Myeloma (Bone Marrow Cancer), a non curable, cancerous disease. So much to take in and we had a wedding to attend in the New Forest. Broke the news to Julie's parents, it's her father's birthday, some present!

Although the disease can not be cured, the patient can be placed in remission from the effects of the condition by the use of strong toxins, generally known as chemotherapy. The method used to place me in remission was a chemical cocktail of carcinogenic drugs called Vincristine, Adriamycin and Dexamethasone (VAD) which are very severe and the treatment can cause the patient further and ongoing problems such as renal failure or becoming diabetic, I suffered both of these conditions, albeit of a temporary nature. The older one becomes, the chances of being given the full strength treatment, is reduced because it is so invasive and potentially harmful. I was 54 when I was diagnosed which is unusual, it normally affects older people. Steroids were also prescribed to give me an increased appetite, which is necessary to combat the effect of weight loss which most cancer sufferers encounter. I lost two stone during the initial treatment although it all went back on later. It also made me bloat around the stomach area, which caused discomfort and distorted vision making driving completely out of the question. I was on high dosages of pain killers, the Class 'A' drug, Morphine Sulphate (MST). The effects of the drug can cause drowsiness and had I been involved in a car crash, the insurance company would not have held themselves responsible for the subsequent costs of the repairs or personal liability claims, so driving was out of the question. In addition to the morphine sulphate tablets, I was also taking up to 20ml of liquid morphine at a time, the affects of which were unpleasant and it was as if I was seeing everything through a video recorder. At one time I would see life in fast forward mode and then that would change as if someone had pressed the pause button. For those readers who remember Max Headroom, the cult television programme of the early eighties, I spoke as he did, a video taped voice emanating from a torso which went into spasms of speech. It is not easy keeping track on the world when you are seemingly in a world of your own and on another planet. You know roughly what you want to say but getting the right words out is rather more difficult, they become twisted and generally make no sense at all, no change there then!

My specialist, Dr Roques explained that over the next few days, we would encounter a number of emotions including; anger, bewilderment, sorry, self pity and many more too numerous to mention. Our drive down to Lyndhurst to meet our daughter Emma was a sober one. Not a lot was said during the rather pensive journey down to the New Forest but much was thought, but there were no tears. As I couldn't drive because it would have been uncomfortable to operate the controls of the car, Julie drove the two-week-old BMW down to Hampshire as if she had driven it for years. I sought comfort from the relatively firm support that the seating in German cars give, it helped my back a lot not to be jolted around from side to side like it was on the 700 bus down to Portsmouth Harbour. The wedding was a formal affair, with plenty of pomp and ceremony held at Richard Branson's exclusive hotel, Rhinefield House deep in the heart of the beautiful New Forest. Emma could gauge the mood and asked if all was in order. What could one say, other than we would explain tomorrow? That wasn't good enough for Emma, and the beans were spilled which rather spoilt her day and a few of her good friends', we didn't want to let on about it, but there are some things which you just can't hide no matter how good an actor you are or may have been.

Saturday 23rd May 1998

We didn't want to break the news to our daughter that day, but you can't hide a thing like cancer. Many tears flowed and she regrets being out in Jersey when she could be close to home during this crisis.

On our return to Worthing following the wedding, and after a wait of only a few days, we were advised that Dr Roques' diagnosis was accurate, it was indeed Multiple Myeloma that I was suffering from and that chemotherapy would commence almost immediately. The staff at the day ward at the hospital were wonderful and gave us their precious time in order to explain the process fully and the likely time scale of events to take place. This process was new to us but sadly commonplace to them, they handled the delicate situation with the ultimate degree of dedication and answered any question we wished to raise. But what questions? How does a person with no medical inclination at all, start to ask about something as potentially life-threatening as cancer? There are a number of organisations and societies dedicated to Multiple Myeloma. They produce excellent pamphlets which are informative and help the newly diagnosed patient and their family through this pernicious disease.

Thursday 28th May 1998

Appointment at 11:00 with Dr Bloomfield at Sussex County Hospital, Brighton for Radiotherapy treatment.

Dr Roques had said that a single course of Radiotherapy might help ease my pain considerably and as luck would have it, the radiologist from Brighton's Oncology Clinic was attending an appointment within the hospital at Worthing that very day which made it a relatively straightforward job of getting him to agree to see me in his clinic in Brighton sooner rather than later. On arrival at the oncology department in due course and in a fairly sedated condition, I misheard a nurse say that she would take me down to the "incineration" department to which I replied that seemed a little final and premature! She told me that she had said "the simulation department" it made one of us laugh, but I can't remember which one. The room to which I was escorted, or rather wheeled in yet another hospital chair, held the simulator that is to all intents and purposes a large Black and Decker 'Work-Mate' marked accordingly with all the angles and measurements necessary to allow pin-point accuracy of the radiation beam. I was indelibly marked so that the radiologist could fire the beam at the precise spot. I had one 40 second blast, and lo and behold within a couple of days I began to notice an improvement. The pain was not as severe, I didn't need to drink as much Oramorph to relieve it. I was advised that I may suffer from some side effects, similar to sunburn or even nausea, but I was very fortunate and didn't experience either of those two symptoms although I know for a fact that some of the other patients in our 'Cancer Club' have experienced a great deal of discomfort.

Sunday 31st May 1998

Admitted to Worthing Hospital in preparation of the Hickman Line being inserted the next day at 14:00 hrs.

I had an antiseptic bath to cleanse my skin of bacteria. There is a very handy system used to deliver the drugs necessary for treatment and also to withdraw blood for analysis, it is via a plastic tube inserted through an opening in the chest and threaded into the Superior Vena Cava, a main artery in the heart. There are two tubes within the Hickman line called lumens, one inside the other and each is capable of being used at the same time for either taking blood or delivering medication. It is a very convenient system, for without it, veins would need to be tapped every time a drug was infused, or blood cultures taken. There is however a price to pay for this convenience, and that is the constant battle against infection in the line. The body knows that the line is an alien being and does its best to get rid of it by rejection. Consequently, a very regular check on my body temperature was undertaken to monitor if a potential problem is developing, I lost two lines through infections but managed to keep the third in long enough for my stem cell transplant in Hammersmith Hospital. The less exposure to possible infection the better and hospitals are renowned for being breeding places for the type of infections that would have been detrimental to my health. Therefore the flushing of my Hickman line was conducted at home by my wife Julie. She was trained in the procedure by the Staff Nurse on the Day Ward and was extremely proficient at it despite the fact that it consumed a great deal of time and meticulous hygiene, which we vigorously adhered to. At one point it was mentioned that a District Nurse could undertake the flushing, but subsequently when one came to visit us, she informed us that she was not qualified to do so as she had not received the correct training!

Thursday 4th June 1998

Starting first dose of chemotherapy at 12:00 in day ward. Will be hooked up to the bum bag containing the VAD fluid so that my heart will act as the pump to get the chemotherapy coursing through my veins.

Today, my visit to the day ward saw the first of six infusions of a toxic poison comprising two chemicals of Vincristine and Doxomocin, collectively known as VAD. It comes in a small bulb shaped dispenser, rather like the bulb on a perfume atomiser and connected to the Hickman line via an extremely fine tube delivering no more than just a drop at a time, over the next five days the chemotherapy would seep, very slowly through the line and into my blood stream. A small bum-bag was worn to contain the VAD bulb and it was practically undetectable in use and had to be kept dry at all costs. After three days, the effect of the chemotherapy started to kick in. I felt sick, very sick and had a distinctly metallic taste in the mouth. Anti-sickness pills helped, but didn't rid me of the nausea symptoms totally. Whilst the chemotherapy was being administered, I was also prescribed steroids, Dexamethazone, these made me ravenously hungry and the fridge was the target of many a mid-night raid. When I was an inpatient at the hospital I would order a plate of sandwiches in addition to my evening meal and place them in the 'fridge in the nurse's kitchen and devour them with relish (or brown sauce if I didn't have any relish!) at 2 A.M. in the morning. By offering to make the night staff a cup of tea, I had an excuse to be in their canteen.

Monday 15th June 1998

Attend day ward to have wound stitches out from Hickman Line and line flush. My hair started to fall out following the commencement of the chemotherapy, it was inevitable and necessitated my bedclothes and pyjamas being changed frequently. It hadn't all fallen out and would have looked better if it had as I looked as if I was suffering from scurvy.

Thursday 18th June 1998

Attended day ward at 10:00 for line flushing, followed by appointment with Dr Roques in his clinic at 11:30. Got telephone call at home at 18:00 to pack a bag and be admitted to hospital.

It appeared that the blood samples taken at clinic earlier in the day had revealed a problem with my kidneys caused by the chemotherapy. I was connected to a saline drip which over the next 48 hours may flush my kidneys out. The following day, the urologist examined me and did an ultrasound test to establish if there was any permanent damage, which fortunately there wasn't. I was urged to drink as much fluid as possible to restore my kidneys to full function, it took a great deal of concerted effort to consume three litres, and sleep patterns were disturbed because of constantly having to get up during the night, still better that than a kidney transplant. Feeling just a little sorry for myself, as the sun's shining and I should have been down in Poole harbour this coming weekend sailing around with my buddy in one of our dinghies. You get used to disappointments and plans changing at relatively short notice. There will be other opportunities, but not this coming weekend. I was discharged on Friday 26th June 1998.

Monday 29th June 1998

Temperature up a bit and feeling unwell, feeling bruised internally from peeing so much. Urologist had a second look at me, all ok, temperature falling from 38°.

Wednesday 1st July 1998

Temperature shot up to 40°, not good news. Trying to stay well today as my sister Pauline is flying down form Norfolk to see me. I am shaking uncontrollably when she arrives. Been given Pethidine as muscle relaxant to stop the shakes.

The tennis at Wimbledon was on the television and I was trying very hard to keep well and look as if there wasn't a problem for when my sister Pauline arrived. How do you tell someone that you're not as bad as you look when you shake with every fibre of your body? She was very concerned about her little brother. I got moved from the general ward into a cubicle at 21:00, which was much quieter for me. With all due respects to my fellow patients, or inmates as I have always referred to them, a general ward of six men, mostly elderly, is like being in a farmyard. The noise of grunting and belching throughout the night makes sleep almost impossible, not to mention the smells that permeate throughout the ward. There was much less chance of an infection being picked up when I was in a room of my own, I only had to be concerned about the good people visiting me in my cubicle, of which there were many. Those with colds would know not to enter, but on a general ward anyone could enter and spread all kinds of germs. I was advised that I could start chemotherapy again on the Friday of that week. I had observed from my penthouse suite's window, the flat roof of the canteen opposite. It was like most other flat roofs, constructed with felt and layered with bitumastic on top of which small stone chippings were scattered to dissipate the heat from the sun. A seagull had laid an egg on the stone chippings, no nest, just a single egg. It was perfectly camouflaged and barely detectable, I knew it was there because I watched the mother gull lay it and constantly tend it. I was in that particular room long enough to see the egg hatch and the chick left on its own whilst its mother was off catching fish for it. Father of course was no where to be seen, he was off with the other boy gulls down the beach or having aerial combats with the crows. Invariably though, they would sit on top of the gasometer adjacent to the hospital, maybe a hundred at a time, all facing the same way in order that their feathers are not ruffled by the breeze, pointing into wind for an easier take off with one small jump. The seagull chick, like the egg it had emerged from, was almost undetectable. I watched it grow and finally take its first faltering 'flight', a vertical jump of six inches with wings flapping wildly, exercising them ready for the time that they would allow him to soar on the thermals coming off the roof. I felt an empathy with the gull, just like Richard Bach's Jonathan Livingstone Seagull. On any return visit to the hospital, I would look at the roof and see my adolescent gull with its brown juvenile feathers, they were slowly turning white like those of his parents, he was also the same size as them and could perform the same aerial manoeuvres. He would come and sit on my window ledge and look in at me, my wife Julie says that he was saying, "Do you remember me?" He could now empathise with me, for he was free and I was the one huddled up in the corner of my 'safe' environment waiting to be fed, sometimes even with fish!

Friday 3rd July 1998

Chemo all set up and ready to start, and then Dr Roques halts the proceedings. He says my blood cultures have revealed a yeast in my blood. Intravenous antibiotics given which caused another rigour, so more pethidine given to stop the quivers.

I told the Doctors a week ago that I could taste yeast in my body and that I felt as if I was fermenting from the inside. This was not the first time that doctors have had to take notice of my explanation that something is not right with my body. Eventually they listened to me and found that I was indeed growing a yeast culture and had to have more antibiotics to cure the problem.

Sunday 5th July 1998

The National Health Service is 50 years old today! We patients are given a special lunch reflecting war time austerity. Carrot pie and heavy puddings to fill us up.

Tuesday 7th July 1998

Not good news, Hickman line infected and must be removed. Despite all their efforts to save the line, the infection had taken hold and was making me ill, I was experiencing a high temperature and the entry site around my Hickman line was inflamed and very sore. A Sister on the day ward removed it under local anaesthetic on Wednesday and even more saline was infused through a canular in my arm to hydrate me. I was discharged on Friday 10th July 1998 with the usual supply of penicillin and antibiotics in case any air borne infections had entered the wound whilst the line was being removed. At a later date I met the Sister's husband at the local swimming pool and showed him his wife's handiwork, "Look" I said, "Your wife attacked me with a knife!" which made the other males in the changing room sit up and take notice.

Sunday 12th July 1998

Julie's "significant" birthday, I'm glad to be home for it. A small gathering had been invited to attend tea at our house in the afternoon by way of a celebration for my wife. Our daughter Emma had now transferred permanently from Jersey to Chichester in order that she could keep her eye on me a little more easily, she felt too remote before and subsequently became a very frequent visitor to my bedside, whether it be at home or in Worthing Hospital.

Sunday 19th July 1998

Admitted to hospital for new Hickman Line to be inserted tomorrow. So another antiseptic bath is called for to cleanse me of external bacteria. On arrival at Worthing Hospital, I made my way up to the fourth floor to Erringham ward and was put into cubicle four again, with the operation to re-insert a new Hickman line due to be conducted on Monday in order that the chemotherapy could recommence on the Tuesday of that forthcoming week.

The operation was a fairly routine procedure and I was back in my bed within a couple of hours of going into theatre. I was a little sore and didn't want anything to eat at meal times, but apart from that I was all right. The next day the doctors deemed that I was well enough to start the chemotherapy treatment again, I attended the day ward and was connected up to the chemotherapy bulb and discharged the same day wearing my now familiar bum bag. I had to attend the day ward on the following Saturday for the VAD to be disconnected and the Hickman lines flushed. It's a little like a publican having to flush the beer pump through in his cellar, if you don't do it to the pipes they become tainted and blocked which is what would happen to my line if it wasn't flushed regularly.

Sunday 26th July 1998

Temperature has risen to 38.1°, rang hospital, they readmitted me. Another problem with the Hickman Line, it's blocked and will not yield blood for analysis. I had only been at home for a week when my temperature started to rise, I knew the rules, if my temperature rose above 38° I was to tell the hospital immediately and if it went up to 38. 5° I was to pack a bag and get myself into hospital as soon as possible.

The nurses have access to a specially formulated liquid, a little like 'Drain-O' which they squirt into the line and leave it for an hour. This generally does the trick and everything is back to normal, or what passes for normal in a cancer patient. With my temperature down again and the line yielding blood for analysis there was no need for me to 'bed block' and was discharged from hospital on Wednesday 29th, with the line saved again. The pain in my back was not too bad and I was not taking as much of the orally administered Oramorph, I also reduced the dosage of the slow release Morphine Sulphate tablets (MST) to just 1 x 10mg pill at night. My sister and brother-in-law had flown down from Norfolk in their aeroplane to see me. Julie collected them from Shoreham Airport, only a mile from our house and five miles from Worthing Hospital. This really was a "flying visit", on that occasion they saw me in better health, not too racked with pain and not shaking uncontrollably. My sister had made a corned beef hash for me as I only wanted to eat simple foods, nothing too heavily flavoured or spiced.

Tuesday 11th August 1998

Attended day ward for third session of chemotherapy (VAD), should be finished by Friday 14th. A bit anaemic, may need blood transfusion. Pain in back still niggling. Able to walk short distances.

Without the encumbrance of the chemo bum bag and with the sun shining brightly, It was time to get out and about for a while. We visited our friends, Graham and his wife, who ran a tea shop on the outskirts of Lewes in East Sussex and spent a pleasant couple of hours with them making deep inroads into their home made cake selection which fuelled me up for a gentle walk on some common land near to them outside a village at Chailey, nothing too strenuous as I was still a little week and wobbly but determined to do it if I possibly could as you can never be sure as to when the opportunity to get out and about will cease.

Monday 24th August 1998

Back pain not being covered by low dose MST, having to increase dose. Appointment with day ward 11:00 for antibiotics.

With the weather being good and still with the desire and ability to get out of the house for a while, we went with our good friends to the West Sussex city of Chichester and had a pleasant pub lunch near the marina in the harbour. There is a delightful harbourside village near to Chichester called Itchenor from which my friend and I had sailed our dinghies on many occasions. However as sailing was completely out of the question at that time, we did what all the visitors do, and took the commercially operated harbour tour on board a 40' motor cruiser, an hour and a half was just enough to feel that you've had an outing and was quite a different experience being able to sail in a straight line rather than having to tack across the main channel to get anywhere. The following day, we met our daughter and partner at another Sussex beauty spot just outside Arundel, known as Swanbourne Lake in the lee of the castle and the South Downs. There is a path of about two miles running around the lake, which I managed to walk with the aide of my trusty hiking pole brought back from a continental holiday one year. This stick, has on more than one occasion, been my only means of support whilst walking or even getting up out of a chair. I couldn't get out of bed at one time without it, I doubt however if I shall need to use the compass built into the top of the stick, but you never know. As I was still feeling all right and not wanting to miss out on any opportunity to take tea out somewhere, we went with my wife's parents to yet another beauty spot, close to Horsham and known as Leonardlee Gardens. There are ornamental lakes to walk around and terraces of Azalea bushes, if you are very fortunate, you get to see the wild wallabies, although on this occasion we didn't and saw only rabbits of which there must be hundreds all nibbling away at the young shoots and plants.

Tuesday 1st September 1998

Have to attend Dr Roques' clinic today in order for a Bone Marrow Biopsy to be conducted.

The procedure is very painful unless you are knocked out, which I now demand to be. The hip is drilled into with a hollow needle which represents a small hand auger and the soft bone marrow is withdrawn for analysis. No matter how robust the blood count may be, it is this biopsy that really reveals whether the cancer is still active or held in check, it is the 'acid test' so to speak. You are drowsy for a couple of hours afterwards and can't drive so the patient always has to have a minder with them. Apparently, and this is only hear say, I had been known to swear at the doctor whilst the needle was going in, but as I was unconscious I had no recollection of it. Following the procedure, a hefty dressing is applied which mustn't become wet for a while and it always seems to be that wooden chair backs are positioned so as to correspond with the wound, which made sitting up to the table for meals rather uncomfortable for a couple of days.

The local airport at Shoreham-by-Sea had its air show today, Saturday 6th September and I felt well enough to attend but I had to be driven there in order to have a base to return to when feeling tired. At one time I was forced into using a wheelchair to give me mobility and the disabled parking scheme's Orange Badge was applied for, this ensured that we had a parking space close to the "flight line" enabling us to enjoy a good view of all the aerial activities.

Monday 7th September 1998

Appointment to attend day ward for 4th session of VAD chemotherapy. Norwich & Norfolk hospital were phoned and an enquiry was made to see if they can disconnect and flush by Friday.

We decided to visit my sister in Norfolk, she had a new "relatives suite" built onto the farmhouse and we were able to stay there. Soon there would not be the chance to travel around, so I took advantage of every opportunity to do so whilst it was available to me. However, no trips were allowed in their aeroplane just in case altitude affected the chemotherapy pump. I was a little disappointed, especially as it was my birthday but understood the reason behind the decision. Whilst we were staying up in East Anglia we had a very busy few days, starting with lunch at

Lowestoft in a café which my sister and brother-in-law frequent for egg and chips and consider it to be quite decadent, followed by a trip around a moored fishing trawler which is now a floating museum.

On another occasion we drove to North Norfolk and finished off the day with tea and dainty sandwiches in a hotel in Blakeney Point overlooking mud flats and further out to sea, a seal colony. We were miles from anywhere, and there out of nowhere were the ubiquitous Japanese tourists with their cameras clicking away at mud flats. The area is, or certainly was when I was a child full of samphire or sea asparagus beds.

Friday 11th September 1998

Appointment 15:00 Weybourne Ward of Norwich & Norfolk Hospital for chemo disconnection and line flush.

It had previously been agreed and arranged by my specialist in Worthing that I could have the chemotherapy bulb disconnected and the line flushed whilst we were up in Norfolk. We met up at the Norwich and Norfolk Hospital in Norwich with my younger nephew, James who was a ward clerk at the time, I received personal treatment, as you would expect and visited the hospital's coffee shop to recover from the terrible ordeal of being pampered. At dinner that same evening my sister stated that "As you've been dodging about here, there and everywhere over the last couple of days, you are either not as poorly as I thought you were, or you're a good actor." The next morning I collapsed on the bathroom floor and that resolved the question of whether or not I was poorly. A frantic telephone call was made to the doctor's surgery and a week-end emergency doctor came to see me within the hour.

Sunday 13th September 1998

Had a very uncomfortable night, feeling of tightness in chest, got up as feeling nauseous and collapsed in bathroom.

Very fortunately the doctor had spent some time in a haematology department and knew all about the effects of my condition and the fact that my white blood cells would be low from the effects of the chemotherapy, which caused me to faint. I was advised to stay in bed all morning, just in case I collapsed again, especially as my temperature was a little higher than is considered normal. We were advised by the doctor that I may need to be admitted to the hospital in Norwich if my temperature didn't moderate. I took dissolvable Paracetamol tablets to bring my temperature down as I didn't really want to be stuck up in a Norfolk hospital with Julie having to drive twenty miles each way to see me. Therefore we decided to make a run for it the next day, if I had to go into hospital, it should be our local hospital in Worthing as they knew everything about me. We got home on Monday tired and exhausted, but at least we were home and could monitor my temperature very closely.

Tuesday 15th September 1998

The inevitable happened, my temperature didn't moderate, so I was readmitted to Worthing Hospital. I have an infection, hopefully not in Hickman Line. Given Intravenous antibiotics of Timentin and Gentamicin, or 'G and T' as it is now affectionately known. Got to stay in hospital until infection clears up, if it ever does.

I was still in hospital on the Sunday of that week and feeling so much better, my temperature was down to an acceptable level and my appetite was restored which is why I escaped with a fellow patient to the canteen and had a cooked breakfast. We had been salivating at the thought of one for several days, and today we made our break for freedom against soggy Weetabix and prunes. The following is a 'tongue in cheek' article I wrote immediately following the event and is entitled;

'The Hospital Egg'

There comes a time during any hospital patient's stay, that the thought of yet another breakfast comprising; soggy cornflakes, undercooked toast and cold tea, is just too much to bear. The body and the mind starts to have cravings for a high cholesterol cooked breakfast with all the trimmings! These cravings were discussed with another 'in-mate' who concurred with me that nothing would set us so well as bacon and eggs. We dressed in our 'civvies' and told the ward sister that 'We're just popping to the canteen for 10 minutes'. No further questions were asked, and no further information given. This could have been our last opportunity and it had to be grabbed. We concealed our hospital identity tags as best we could under our pullovers and attempted to look like ordinary visitors to the canteen. On arrival we helped ourselves to the various fat-laden breakfast foods, being careful to avoid the cereals and fresh fruit. To our dismay, there were only scrambled eggs on display, so I asked the chef who was in attendance, 'Could I have two fried eggs please?' To which the reply came, 'Fried eggs are not available, we only have scrambled'. With my heart set on a fried egg, I enquired if instead of breaking the eggs and scrambling them, why can't he just crack one and fry it? The answer came, 'These eggs have been irradiated to be a more healthy option for the patient.' The fact that the scrambled eggs were soft and runny and could have contained salmonella poisoning because of it, held no defence in the eyes of the chef. 'So what if you just crack open an irradiated egg and not scramble it?' was my retort. 'No can't do that,' came his reply, 'you see we buy them in from our suppliers all ready scrambled and just heat 'em through,' he advised me. Very hygienic I thought. Instead of a hermetically sealed sack contained within a hard coated shell (admittedly out of a chicken's bottom!), I would have to have re-heated, pre-bought, irradiated and scrambled eggs. He was adamant that it was not possible to supply fried eggs, so I gave in and settled for scrambled eggs. The next morning, having enjoyed the previous day's breakfast, albeit with no fried egg, I presented myself to the breakfast buffet to be met by a different chef, I smiled, said 'good morning' and proceeded to help myself to his scrambled eggs, not even daring to ask the same question as yesterday. 'Good morning' came his reply, 'Would you like a fried egg with that breakfast'? I could have kissed him! Tale Ends.

Later that day, I was moved into cubicle six on Erringham ward where my wife Julie was provided with a camp bed and she stayed that night with me as I was due to go up by hospital car service to Hammersmith Hospital to see the haematology specialist the following day.

Monday 21st September 1998

We would get to learn of the options available to me for my Bone Marrow Transplant and the potential mortality rate for each. Doctor Apperley told my wife and self that an autograft uses my own stem cells and during treatment there is only a 5% chance of death, whereas an allograft uses the stem cells from a donor and carries a 20% chance of death. These were hard facts, put to us in a no nonsense manner. When confronted with a choice as stark as that, the only option we could have possibly taken was to have an autograft using my own stem cells. Got back to Worthing Hospital and told that the infection in the Hickman Line is too virulent and the line must be removed tomorrow.

Tuesday 22nd September 1998

The ward Sister removed my line under local anaesthetic by cutting the flesh around the entry site and simply pulling the line out. It didn't hurt and there was no bleeding. Discharged same day with yet another patch stuck on me. Later that week we met up with friends to enjoy a cup of tea and a cake at a riverside café in Amberley near Arundel, I couldn't go inside for fear of picking up another infection which would have delayed me receiving further treatment for a while which had to avoided at all costs because of the importance of the being given the transplant to hold the disease in check.

I had this notion that as I would be in hospital at Hammersmith for anything up to a month whilst receiving my treatment, that I would need something to occupy my mind, so with the same friends we went to Dorking for lunch a few days later and I attended an open day for the Open University making enquiries about some sort of study course that I could undertake, however they wanted 'proper money' for it and I didn't take up their offer. During that same week, the tall brick chimney of the old power station in Shoreham was to be demolished by being blown up in a blaze of publicity. The local newspaper had run a competition to see who would be the lucky person who got to detonate the explosion, it was won by Leon, a fellow cancer sufferer whom I'd met in the day ward at the hospital on a few occasions. We had swapped experiences such as; when and where did he have his allograft, how inclined was he to use his laptop computer during the time he was in isolation at the hospital etc, the answer to my question was that he just didn't feel well enough and therefore didn't use the computer very often. It was just as well that I didn't spend proper money on a university course if I wasn't going to be able to concentrate on studying. Sadly, Leon died a short while afterwards but I look at the new chimney at the power station and regard it as a monument to him and the brave manner in which he coped with his Leukaemia.

Monday 12th October 1998

Admitted to Worthing Hospital again for insertion of third Hickman Line. Had Operation at 11:30 next day. Had to stay in for ten days because of infection in urine and a chest infection, got discharged on Thursday 22nd.

Sunday 25th October 1998

Temperature still causing concern, got readmitted. Given intravenous antibiotics of Timentin and Vancamicin to combat the effects of the infection. I am neutropenic (no immunity to infections) and tachicardic (heart beating faster than normally) temperature still 38°

Friday 6th November 1998

Temperature rising to 38.2°, had to advise hospital who want me to report in. I hope there is not an infection in this new Hickman line already! The very last thing I wanted to happen was for the new line to have become infected so soon after being inserted and if measures could be taken sooner rather than later to save it, then every trick in the book should be used. Blood samples were taken at hospital and analysed straight away but nothing was apparent, so I didn't get admitted. We don't know what caused temperature to 'spike', but it reduced to a reasonable level and the panic was over. The surgeon said he was running out of places in my chest to insert another line so soon after the last one.

Sunday 8th November 1998

Spoke too soon! got phone call from hospital at 18:30, they've found that I do have an infection and I've got to be admitted immediately! Given Vancomicin antibiotic through line, transferred into cubicle 3 at 23:00. Dr Roques says I can go home tomorrow after third treatment of Vancomicin. I was discharged at 19:00 the following Monday on the promise that I attended the day ward on a daily basis until the 21st of the month for treatment as an outpatient. I was also given Granulocyte Colony Stimulating Factor (GCSF) which promotes the growth of cells in the peripheral blood where immature or stem cells are harvested prior to a stem cell transplant. The GCSF is not given via the line, but injected directly into the stomach, it wasn't too uncomfortable. Steroids had bloated my stomach up making the nurses job a little easier, there was plenty to aim at!

Monday 11th November 1998

Collected by hospital car driver at 07:00, going to Hammersmith for heart and lung efficiency tests, x-rays and the all important Stem Cell Harvest etc. The lung capacity test up at Hammersmith Hospital was conducted by a young lady, who obviously had my best interests at heart although at the time it didn't seem like it. I was bullied into exhaling every ounce of breath from my lungs. The process involved placing, what is best described as a vacuum cleaner hose in my mouth, taking a very deep breath in and then exhaling until your eyes pop out of your head. When I waved my arms to indicate that I was on the point of expiration, the reaction I received was that "If you stopped waving your arms about, you would have enough breath to achieve the required reading on the instrument." She was trying to establish that I had sufficient lung capacity to cope with the treatment before being admitted to hospital for the bone marrow transplant, but it still felt as if I was being bullied. By comparison the cardiogram to establish the condition of my heart, was a pleasant lie down for half an hour with little or no exertion on my behalf. It was two days later that I found the last of the self adhesive tabs that hold the electrodes in place, by that time the adhesive substance had set and it took me another two days to get the glue off my skin.

The process for the extraction of stem cells was an interesting experience, I was connected to what can best be described as an adapted kidney dialysis machine. One set of tubes were connected to my Hickman line and the others to a canula inserted in my arm, this enabled the blood to circulate throughout, both my body and the machine. The sister in charge told me to lie still for three hours, three hours! I don't do that even when I'm asleep. When the colour of my blood matched a sample shown on a colour chart attached to the machine known as Flocytometry (a little like a mix and match paint chart at B&Q), a centrifuge was switched on to withdraw my stem cells which were pale salmon pink in colour and identified by an associated protein numbered CD34. Having established that they had collected sufficient cells from the harvest for the forthcoming treatment and that I was fit enough to receive the stem cell transplant, I was sent home by hospital car and told to await a phone call regarding my admission date, which came through a few days later.

I was admitted on Sunday 27th November 1998. The following chapter explains the procedure involved in the transplant procedure itself and life behind bars for nearly four weeks.

Chapter Three.

The Transplant.

The much-awaited day for my stem cell transplant had arrived, the day we hoped could let us see some light at the end of a very dark tunnel. My transplant was to be an autograft, using my own stem cells that had been harvested on a previous visit to Hammersmith hospital. I was fortunate that the harvest was successful, otherwise an allograft would have to have been conducted using the stem cells from a donor which may not have matched my own and caused me rejection problems. My wife, Julie, and myself were collected from Worthing hospital where I had been an inpatient for the last few days. The hospital car service driver arrived at 10:30 on Sunday the 22nd of November 1998. We were driven to London's Hammersmith Hospital, part of the Imperial College of Medicine where we were both to be for the best part of the next month whilst my treatment was taking place.

Julie had previously been asked if she wanted to stay in my room with me, she accepted as she wanted to see everything first hand and would know how I was feeling rather than me simply saying that 'I was alright,' when I might not have been. We arrived at the hospital in good time and the restaurant was still open for lunch, roast pork was chef's special of the day and it proved to be the only meal that I really appreciated for the next two months. Our belongings, which were quite numerous, were placed into room seven and as no treatment was due to be carried out for the rest of the day, we were free to roam and explore our surroundings. The sun was out, we were full of optimism, so we took ourselves off to see the sights of East Acton, which is not quite the epicentre of architecturally interesting buildings, but at least it wasn't hospital. I made the most of being able to walk around for a while before resigning myself to the fact that I wasn't going to set foot on the pavement again for the next month. On our return to Dacie ward, we were introduced to Gill who was to be my named nurse for the duration of my stay. All the staff are truly dedicated, but Gill was specifically dedicated, or assigned to me and would see me more often than any of the other members of the nursing staff. The rest of the day was spent becoming familiar with our surroundings within the hospital and trying to find a fold up bed for Julie that actually worked and didn't collapse as soon as she lay on it to test it. Whilst Julie was in hospital with me, she was able to come and go as she pleased provided that she thoroughly washed her hands and changed out of street clothes, washed her hands with special anti-bacteria soap and applied alcohol gel, donned a blue plastic apron on her return to the ward and that was it! She had to wear a clean set of clothes every time she came back to the hospital and these were washed with mine every day at extremely high temperatures to ensure that no germs were imported into my safe environment.

Hospitals are notorious for being the breeding ground for bugs and diseases such as M. R. S. A. so every precaution had to be taken to avoid me having any problems arising from infections whilst my immune system was suppressed through the use of chemotherapy.

Monday 23rd November 1998

Today is designated as day one in hospital and day minus three to my bone marrow transplant, or stem cell transplant as it is more commonly referred to as it uses different techniques. Blood samples were taken, but no other treatment is due today other than taking tablets to avoid problems with damage to kidneys prior to receiving the high dose chemotherapy, Melphalan through my Hickman line. The day for me was quite unadventurous although I was permitted to walk around inside the main hospital building to buy a newspaper or simply to stretch my legs, I knew that once treatment commenced, this privilege wouldn't last for much longer and I made the most of it.

Tuesday 24th November 1998

Day two in hospital and day minus two to BMT. Having high dosage chemotherapy, Melphalan today, x-ray on my head to ensure there is no undetected metal in my eyes, skull etc. prior to a scan using a Magnetic Resonance Imaging (MRI) scanning device.

Today saw me watching intrigued as Gill, my nurse, hooked me up to a large syringe containing the carcinogenic chemotherapy fluid via my Hickman line. The manner in which it was to be administered had to be very precise and necessitated the container being connected to a pump set to deliver it at a predetermined rate, to exceed the required dosage could have killed me, so every care was taken, checked and double checked. When this was infused I was summoned to go for an MRI scan, questions were asked as to whether I had any metal plates in my head or had ever had metal fragments in my eyes. I said that I once had to have rust from an exhaust pipe removed from the eye. This caused a certain amount of confusion and a porter was sent for to wheel me off to the x-ray department in order that they could check my eyes to ensure that all traces had been removed, which they had. I believe that the radiologist was concerned in case any residual metal gave a false reading on his machine or possibly would have heated up under the scanning process. I imagined it to be similar to the space shuttle crews having to have their teeth fillings drilled out and replaced with ceramic ones because of the heat transference. For a description of a MRI scanning machine, imagine six old Bendix washing machines bolted together and placed in a darkened room with a heavy steel-lined door, there are no windows and the operatives secrete themselves behind an armour-plated glass screen well away from the MRI machine. I felt most ill at ease for the next 40 minutes whilst the machine made thumping sounds as the scanner travelled along its track and lights flashed and flickered intermittently. The fact that I was given an emergency panic button to press did nothing for my confidence or comfort, I mean if they expect you to panic, it must be pretty awful, and it was! The operatives can't tell you that of course because they've never been in one, they just tell you that you'll hear a slight knocking sound. I asked several of the staff members how they knew there would be a slight knocking sound and the reply was "Because we can hear it from here" What they failed to realise was that the sound was being muffled by their glass screen several feet away from the scanner, the patient however hears it all in glorious wraparound sound.

The Melphalan chemotherapy dose of 200mg was so strong that I could begin to taste It and feel its effect within an hour or so of being infused. I was put on a saline drip to ensure sufficient fluids were going through my kidneys as the treatment is hard on them, as is the Multiple Myeloma in itself. Whilst receiving chemotherapy, it was very important to follow the guide lines regarding mouth care, especially as this was one area that could have caused me to have infections as the mouth contains a large number of bacteria. Basically, I was told to sponge cleanse my teeth rather than brushing them so as not to damage the gums and I had to use the prescribed mouth-wash very regularly, it was evil tasting stuff, but it has to be used, it also turned my teeth a dirty brownish colour typical of smokers teeth, except I didn't smoke.

Wednesday 25th November 1998

Day three inside and minus one to receiving my stem cells. Drugs given to combat effect of nausea caused by chemo.

Sadly the drugs to prevent sickness didn't help, I was ill several times during the night, but as I had to get up anyway to pass water every hour because of all the fluids, I was awake and so was Julie. Vomiting means even less fluids are being retained and the saline drip had to continue. I lost the benefit of my slow release morphine tablets (MST), through being ill and couldn't face any food either, the taste of the chemo became all pervading and no food or drink tasted as it should, I was at risk of dehydration if I couldn't ingest sufficient fluids on my own so a glucose drip was connected to my line to hydrate me.

Thursday 26th November 1998

Zero day, I get my stem cells today on forth day of being in hospital. Blood transfusion due and more sickness cover.

My nurse, Gill advised me that when the stem cells were to be reintroduced into my blood stream via the Hickman line, that there would be a certain smell that accompanies the process, which can make a patient feel nauseous. Intrigued, I asked what kind of smell, thinking it to be similar to silage or rotting eggs, however it turned out to be a smell similar to either sweetcorn or oysters which can be quite unpleasant for some patients. Just in case I was affected, scented candles were lit in an attempt to camouflage the smell, but I would have preferred the natural smell of the stem cells, (which in my mind didn't smell at all!) but others in the room can always smell it, much the same as eating garlic, the person eating it can't smell it on their breath, but others can. The transplant was, it must be said, a bit of an anti-climax, a trolley was wheeled in and on it stood a stainless-steel cabinet with dials and buttons on it, straight out of Dr Who. The cells were in the same type of clear plastic bag that patients are given when having a blood transfusion, because to all intents and purposes, that is exactly what it is. The young, pink, blood cells were fed through my Hickman line during the next hour and that was it! No drama, no doctor in a white gown telling me that "When I wake up it will all be over", Gill hooked me up and flushed the line afterwards as if it was a normal blood transfusion, which I also had later on in the day because my red blood cell count had dropped to below the critical figure of ten.

Friday 27th November 1998

Second blood transfusion due on this day plus one since BMT and fifth inside. Also due for Immunoglobulin to help my stem cells grow to boost immune system. The days which took me round to the middle of the following week remained much the same as last week, Feeling nauseous, the pills were catching in my closing throat and my immune system was failing rapidly. Some medication was available in liquid form, however the taste of those made me feel more ill than attempting to swallow the drug in pill form, some drugs could be given via my Hickman line but not all of them. I was starting to feel very poorly and was indeed very poorly, but I also knew that I was on the road to recovery, well partial remission any way.

Thursday 3rd December 1998

Have reached rock bottom now, no immune system (Neutropenic), feeling nauseous all the time, unable to eat or drink, can't keep anything down. Have never felt so ill in my entire life, or certainly these last eleven days in hospital. It is now 7 days since my BMT.

Having reached a neutropenic state because my neutrophils had dropped (a state where I had no immune system at all), I was at risk from picking up infections from three main sources;

[1] My own skin, mouth or organisms in the gut.

[2] Cross infections, i. e. passed on from other people.

[3] Organisms found in my food, such as Salmonella etc.

Normally, my body's natural defences, generated by the leucocytes would have coped with any infections, but having no defence at all, put me at risk from all sources. Basically my body was trying to kill me, we all have good and bad bacteria in our bodies and in a reasonably healthy person the balance is maintained and no problems arise, but when a person has no defence against bad bacteria, they try to take over and would eventually be very detrimental to health.

Friday 4th December 1998

Now being fed and watered through my Hickman Line because my throat has closed up completely, the technical term being Mucusitis, feels like swallowing glass shards. All the nourishment I needed was contained in the bag of "Total Patient Nourishment"(TPN). The Diamorphine levels have been increased to cover the pain in my throat.

The feeling of pain in my throat from the mucusitis was excruciating to say the least, imagine attempting to swallow broken glass, it was as painful as that, except I couldn't swallow, my mouth was salivating and I had to use a dish to empty my mouth of saliva. Eating and drinking were impossible and had to rely on being given fluids via my Hickman line. The TPN cost £100 a bag and I was getting through three every day, it looked a little like one of the other proprietary build-up drinks that my mother used to feed me with, called Bengers. Goodness knows what was in the TPN because the resulting waste it produced was like something out of Prof. Quatermass and the Pit for those readers old enough to remember yet another cult television programme.

Tuesday 8th December

Day 16 in hospital and 12 days since my BMT. Spiking a temperature, being given antibiotics and put on Oxygen as levels in blood are below 95% of normal. Due also for C. T. (CAT) scan as x-ray shows shadow on my lung. The most recent blood sample revealed that my; White blood cell (Leucocytes which are produced in the bone marrow and designed to kill micro-organisms) count was 0.3, Platelets were 12 and Stem Cells (Neutrophils) 0.12 against an average of 5.6, which indicated that anything higher than zero meant that my immune system was returning slowly but surely.

Typical Normal Blood Counts are;

	White Blood Cells	*Platelets - Red Blood Cells*
Adult Male:	*3.7 to 9.5*	*143 to 332 - 13.2 to 16.7*
Adult Female:	*3.9 to 11.1*	*143 to 332 - 11.8 to 14.8*

Wednesday 9th December 1998

Julie's parents had made the pilgrimage from the south coast by public transport to see me in the knowledge that I could receive visitors again because my immunity was returning. The hospital may be known as Hammersmith Hospital but it is physically located some two miles away in East Acton and not easily reached by direct transport links. Any underground rail passengers alighting at Hammersmith and expecting to find the hospital close by are going to be disappointed. A change is necessary to catch a train to East Acton station which has a very small road frontage and could be missed if you blinked. An easier route by public transport is to catch a tube to White City and then the 75 bus which draws up outside the hospital. Not an easy journey for octogenarians or any one who is non-ambulant. For their return journey they were to be accompanied by my wife who had decided that she would return to our house in Sussex to attend to bills, other mail and to get a change of clothes as her others had been washed to death by the hospital's heavy duty laundry service.

Thursday 10th December 1998

Immune system getting much better as; white blood cell count (WBC) has risen to 1.0, platelets to 29 and neutrophils up to 0.39 from 0.12. Today is 18th day in hospital and 14 since BMT. Doctors pleased with progress, may be out of here next week.

Monday 14th December 1998

Day 18 since BMT and 22nd day in hospital. Getting shakes as Diamorphine reducing, can go home when at zero. I am in what is referred to as 'Cold Turkey' state. WBC count now 3.3 and Platelets at 44, neutrophils gone up to 1.03 and doctors continue to be pleased with progress.

Julie arrived back at hospital by lunchtime following her short stay at home, it gave her a break from being couped up with me in our small room all the time, our friends kindly brought her up from Sussex by car to save her the inconvenience of battling with public transport. Eating still wasn't easy for me, I was only able to eat soft foods such as; yoghurt, custard, rice pudding, soup and jelly. Nothing substantial yet as my throat was still very tender from when it closed up because of the Mucusitis. Once I was able to prove to the doctors that I managed to eat solid foods, I was told that I would go home the next day, however I was still suffering from drug related withdrawal symptoms, the "cold turkey" effect as the pain killer in the Diamorphine pump was now disconnected and I would give a sudden twitch, only once every so often, but it was a violent action which did nothing for my damaged spine. I was attempting to read the Times newspaper and was reading about Nicola Horlick's sad loss of her eldest daughter Georgina to leukaemia, it tended to bring it all home rather and then the newspaper would almost fly out of my hands whilst I was trying to control it. I couldn't go home until I was off the pain killers completely, and having been in hospital for over three weeks, I decided it was better to suffer the odd involuntary shake than go home too soon.

Tuesday 15th December 1998

Very restless night because of withdrawal symptoms, stomach upset. Convinced doctors that I could eat solids and on my 19th day after receiving the BMT, I was allowed home. Had to see dietician regarding what to eat at home.

The day finally came when I could go home, 23 days after being admitted. The hospital's dietician came to see me and discussed various options for a diet that would build up my strength but would not expose me to risk of salmonella poisoning or other food related problems. He was a huge young man and built like a brick bus shelter, probably a rugger player but certainly not one to be messed with even if I felt like it, which I didn't. I was discharged with all the relevant paperwork to give to my specialist at Worthing hospital and GP in Shoreham. There were numerous pills and potions that had to be collected from the pharmacy department which was exceptionally busy and necessitated a forty minute wait for the drugs to be dispensed. We made our way to the patients' waiting room loaded down with suitcases and various bags expecting to be put in a hospital car immediately. However we waited for four hours before a hospital car became available as they always deliver local patients home first and then take outlying patients home later. It was not ideal to be sitting in a communal discharge lounge with people coughing and sneezing all around me, but it was still a better option than risking public transport. Our lift home only happened at all because one of the nurses who had been looking after me saw that I was still in the patients' lounge and went to complain bitterly upon my behalf. We got home to Sussex at 20:30 that night thoroughly exhausted and my legs were aching like crazy. I missed not having my drip stand for support whilst walking and my legs felt very weak, hardly surprising really as I hadn't been anywhere for over a month. Our time was occupied during the following week by reading up all the things that we could, or couldn't do food wise. Each day in hospital a hostess would bring round a menu card enabling the patient to choose their meals for the following day. Invariably there were mince pies or puddings with suet available, but not for me, they were not allowed so I had to have a yoghurt or rice pudding. Christmas was but a few days away, and I wasn't allowed any of the usual trappings, such as sausage-meat stuffing, Christmas pudding or anything like that. We were invited to our friends for Christmas Day lunch and special instructions had to be given as to what I was entitled to eat and what I was not, it was quite onerous on the host but she managed admirably. This regime of careful dietary control lasted for approximately four weeks until it was considered that my immune system had been restored and that I was in partial remission.

ALLOWED TO EAT:

Breakfast Cereals:	Could only be from individual packs and once opened could not be saved for another occasion, so the small individual cereal packets were a godsend.
Cheese:	Individually wrapped portions of hard or processed cheese, soft varieties allowed only if made from Pasteurised milk. Yoghurt: Pasteurised yoghurt only.
Eggs:	Must be well cooked (fear of Salmonella poisoning).
Meat:	Must be freshly cooked not raw, the same applies to fish.
Vegetables:	Fresh or freshly cooked from frozen only.
Fruit:	All fruit must be peeled.
Sweets:	Individually wrapped sweets and chocolate were permitted.
Puddings:	Tinned fruit but not saved over from another day, individually wrapped ice cream, tinned rice pudding,
Drinks:	Carbonated water and soft drinks if individually bottled. Chemically produced beer.

NOT ALLOWED:

Live Yoghurt:	Ones with active bacteria in, i.e. Bio-yoghurt.
Certain Cheeses:	Stilton, Brie, Dolcelatta, Camembert and Gorgonzola.
Shell Fish:	Not allowed.
Meat:	No pates or processed meats.
Puddings:	No mince pies or Christmas pudding (contains suet).
Drinks:	No real ale or live yeast culture beer, no still bottled water, tap water has to be boiled before use.
Miscellaneous:	No pepper.

Getting back to normal.

One of the first experiences ex-patients feel when they are discharged from hospital is sheer exhaustion. The inactivity over the last four weeks or so meant that muscle tissue had wasted away and needed gentle exercise to rebuild it. Although most wards had an exercise bike, for much of the time the patient is either neutropenic and can't leave the confines of their room to use it, or have very little inclination to do so anyway because of feeling too poorly.

The outside world also appeared so huge to me after the confines of a twelve foot square room and the pace at which traffic travelled was quite frightening. It took several weeks after my discharge before I felt able to cope with the driving experience again. It was good to see that some of the trees were in leaf, a bit of colour in my world that had previously been totally dominated by magnolia painted walls. When the interior of our house was to be repainted, it would be in any colour other than magnolia, I'd overdosed on it and that was the very last colour I wanted to sit and look at!

Some patients have pets at home, so special care is needed to avoid any problems whilst white blood cells are still low and the immune system yet to be fully restored. Ideally, someone else should groom and feed a family pet, which is also to be discouraged from being in close proximity to food preparation areas and sleeping arrangements but these are common sense precautions anyway and most people don't need telling of the obvious, but the hospital wanted to ensure that all patients were aware of the potential risks involved. Although to 'pet' an animal is soothing and does much to aid the recovery of the patient, care should be exercised in allowing the animal to lick the hands and face of the patient in case germs are transmitted. Although this is common sense, it pays to be diligent in hygiene and general matters of cleanliness throughout the house.

Friday Christmas Day 1998

Doesn't feel much like Christmas Day, I'm thin having lost two stone, I'm cold because I've no hair at all and fatigued because my muscles have wasted away.

Our friends very kindly bought me a Christmas present of woollen hat to wear and our host stuck religiously to our dictates as to the quirks of my diet. I hadn't had any alcohol at all for about eight weeks, apart from the mouth wash prescribed by the hospital which tasted awful and is only good for spitting out as you are intended to do. Others, I understand do drink it, but you would have to be really desperate. I had a small amount of Liebfraumilch wine topped up with lemonade, and managed to spill it in my freshly cooked roast turkey dinner, I stuck to drinking Appletise after that. Later in the day I began to feel quite tired and went home after we had a light tea of tinned fruit salad and condensed milk with bread and spread. It rather reminded me of the teas we used to have whilst I was living at home as a youngster with my parents. The rest of that week was fairly uneventful, no dramas on the health front and I was continuing to regain my strength and appetite to some degree albeit rather slowly but I was home and that made me feel much better just being in my own surroundings.

Thursday New Year's Eve 1998

New Years Eve, got to go to Hammersmith for check up and removal of Hickman line.

The hospital must have been satisfied that I was doing all right following my transplant, otherwise they wouldn't have removed my line. When I'd had the two previous lines removed at Worthing, it was under a local anaesthetic and the Dacron cuff which is designed to knit with the soft tissue underneath the skin, was cut away by a Sister who subsequently sewed the wound up to prevent infection. However, a diminutive, female Chinese doctor advised me she was going to remove my line, I therefore thought nothing of it when she picked up the line, assuming that it was because she wished to examine the entry wound. Not a bit of it!, with one swift tug, the line was out. "What about the Dacron cuff that's designed to prevent the line being pulled out inadvertently, I asked" when my composure had been regained. "Oh it's alright, that stays in your chest as the line slipped through the middle of it" The cuff is about the same size and shape of a Polo mint, which I can never eat without making the direct comparison.

I didn't see the New Year in, I was far too exhausted. I didn't even toast the occasion, being abstinent from alcohol for so long, it would have made me ill immediately. I was now at home, very weak and susceptible to picking up colds and 'flu. It was recommended that I didn't go on public transport, fly or go in shops for the next six weeks. Suited me because I didn't feel up to doing any of that anyway! So with the exception of visiting either, Worthing or Hammersmith hospitals for the next six weeks, I didn't do a great deal. Numerous friends and family wanted to visit, each had to be vetted for coughs and colds, they still are.

My diet for the next four weeks, was very closely monitored, not because of weight, but for suitability of ingredients. It was ages before I could catch up on the missed mince pies, but I did eventually, and thoroughly enjoyed them when I was able. The time came when I was able to get out and about, visit friends who would drag me off to the pub and attempt to ply me with real ale. I should have enjoyed it, but when you've been without it all for so long, you can't cope with it. I did eventually learn to do so of course, but initially it was all too much for me. I was deemed to be in remission, a statement that was music to my ears being a cancer patient. I could consider continental travel once more as my insurance company were prepared to reinstate my cover, and I would try and lead a life that was near to 'normal' as possible. I couldn't however return to work for a number of reasons including; back pain when carrying computers, the opiate-based drugs to stem the pain in my back would have nullified any motor insurance cover, and the constant exposure to life threatening infections caught from my clients or their children was also a deciding factor.

An enquiry was made of the specialist as to how long I could expect to remain in remission, and was told, "There are no hard and fast rules with your condition, it's not a curable disease and an average period of time in remission is approximately thirty months." It was truly amazing how such a finite number of months could be quoted for a remission period. The hospital however are accustomed to treating diseases such as mine and knew from past experience, how long an average period in remission was likely to be. This turned out to be uncannily accurate. From the information given to me by the specialists, I knew that for the next two and a half years, I could expect to have a reasonable quality of life and I should get out and about as much as possible for you never know when these activities will cease. The disease had softened my spine and eaten into the vertebrae, making the bones porous and brittle, therefore, taking into consideration my condition and making sure that I did not place myself in a position of jeopardy, like hang gliding or bungee jumping, there would be no reason why I should not enjoy the next thirty months and regain some quality of life. There was however the feeling that the situation could change at any time without warning and that my period of time in remission would be over sooner rather than in two and a half years time. Therefore, the Sword of Damocles was constantly above my head and was waiting to fall at any time and without any given notice. I strongly recommend to anyone placed in the same position that I was in, to travel now, for tomorrow may be too late. If the patient feels reasonably well enough to travel and knowing that there has to be a time when that ability ceases, don't put it off, do it now because there may not be another opportunity. Obviously it is down to the individual and their medical advisers who should have the last word and decide if travel to a certain destination is feasible, if it is and you want to go. The same criteria applies to hobbies and pastimes, if you have a yearning to take up an interest, do it. Bear in mind your own capabilities and competency, but go and do it now, for as with travelling you may not get a second chance, life's too short. I used to sail quite frequently, right up to the time I was diagnosed. Strangely enough the fluid motion of the boat through the water was quite comfortable for me, more so in fact than the car journey to where the boat was kept. I experienced some back pain, but didn't let it stop me initially as I thought I would soon be over the muscle strain that the local GP had diagnosed. It helped quite considerably having my sailing buddy, Alan, who would help drag the sailing dinghy up the ramp from the water and erect the mast if it were necessary.

Monday 11th January 1999

Got collected at 08:30 by hospital car service for check up at Hammersmith. They need to know that my autograph has taken and that my immunity is coming back. Still in pain from myeloma and taking slow release morphine tablets, MST.

Thursday 14th January 1999

"Flying visit" from my sister and brother-in-law from Norfolk. Julie collected them from Shoreham airport. They brought numerous gifts of food and drink to encourage me to eat and gain weight as I have lost two stones.

Tuesday 19th January 1999

The dietician from Hammersmith rang to say I can revert to a normal diet now, just over a month since being discharged from hospital. Still taking MST for back pain as still giving me a disturbed night.

Because I was feeling so much better and had regained some weight and strength, it was time to consider booking a holiday. We had to cancel last year's due to my illness and hospitalisation and we hoped for more success this year. We hoped to travel to the lakes of northern Italy which is one of our favourite destinations and in particular, Lake Maggiore. July was to be our chosen time to travel as by then my general health was considered to be so much better and my strength returned enabling me to cope with the rigours of air travel.

Thursday 4th February 1999

Busy day, due at day ward for another infusion of the bone strengthening agent, Pamidronate and then to have a bone marrow biopsy, for which I will be sedated.

Monday 8th February 1999

Another check up at Hammersmith, being collected by hospital car service at 08;15, It's cold outside and there is frost on the roads.

All must have been well up at Hammersmith, for after my bloods were taken and analysed they announced that I didn't need to go for another check up for three months. Three whole months of being able to travel and get out and about, sheer bliss. I was invited by a friend, David, to attend an exhibition at Olympia London. He had a stand at a trade show for the travel industry and said I could be a 'Stand Dolly' sitting and watching the world go by, talking to the occasional person and accepting free glasses of champagne when offered. It was good to get into a business environment again, although I played no part in the proceedings.

Thursday 25th February 1999

Not quite given a free hand to travel anywhere I wished as got to see Dr Roques in Worthing today. Having blood test, white blood cells (infection-fighting cells) were imbalanced, he wants to check that I'm OK.

Because of suffering no ill effects from my last trip to London with my friend, David had invited me again to another trade show which took place at Earls Court London on the following Monday, it was tiring, but enjoyable. I managed to stay out of trouble health wise at any rate. The train journey was only an hour and a half so not too onerous on me.

Thursday 25th March 1999

A month after the last visit to his clinic, Dr Roques wants to check on my blood count etc. I need to collect a further supply of pills and potions.

Thursday 1st April 1999

More Pamidronate to strengthen bones, due at 10:00 in day ward. Asked about an injection against catching Shingles (Herpes Zoster) as Julie's mother has it.

Sunday 4th April 1999

Day ward for injection against Herpes Zoster, can't be too careful. I wonder how long the protection lasts?

Tuesday 13th April 1999

Feeling very good today, no side effects from medication and back pain is tolerable, may be able to consider resuming work again shortly if good health holds up, it's nearly a year since I was diagnosed. Due to see Dr Roques again on 22nd. April.

Tuesday 27th April 1999

Due at day ward in Worthing today for more Pamidronate and another bone marrow biopsy, will be knocked out for a couple of hours again.

As I was still feeling quite good, Julie and myself decided to visit relatives in Norfolk. My sister and brother-in-law had extended an invitation to us, so we went whilst the opportunity existed. There are pleasant walks over two local golf courses close to their property and as the sun was shining, we took advantage of them both. My sister had 'grounded' me from flying last time we visited because I was hooked up to my chemotherapy pouch, now that I wasn't connected to the pump I was able to fly in my brother-in-law's aeroplane. Very convenient when it's hangared in a barn on the farm land they own adjacent to their house. On our return to Sussex, my former boss at the insurance company had written ask for an appointment to see me. She wanted to discuss the possibility, or as it turned out, impossibility of returning to work and offered an invalidity pension to retire me early. I was 55 and hadn't considered retiring so early, but accepted the situation that with my medical condition it would be difficult for me to work to a normal pattern and would always have the need to take time off for medical appointments and treatment.

I had just started to read John Diamond's "C" Because Cowards get Cancer and could empathise with him over several elements of his illness. John's wife was Nigella Lawson of cooking and being a domestic goddess fame. John later died from cancer of the tongue.

Monday 10th May 1999

The three-monthly appointment at Hammersmith requires me to be there by 11:00. The hospital car came for us both at 08:45. Due to see Dr Apperley following blood checks to ensure that all is as it should be, very protective towards patients who have had bone marrow transplants. All satisfactory, can travel to Geneva on Monday as planned.

Monday 17th May 1999

I travelled to another trade show in Geneva with the same friend, he needed the moral support and someone to organise him. Despite all my efforts to do so, he misplaces his passport, our plane tickets and the hotel reservation confirmation. I thought of starting to walk back home to Sussex from Heathrow airport at that point, it would have been less stressful. Subsequently we were late getting to the airport and missed our flight but British Airways put us on a later flight via Zurich. We had a couple of hours to kill but that is insufficient time to go anywhere or see anything so our time was spent in the executive lounge getting our fill of Danish pastries, coffee and Brandy. We eventually arrived safely and that evening in Geneva where there was a violent thunder storm, I think someone high and mighty may be telling him something. The weather generally in Geneva in the Spring is wonderful and this year was no exception. Although the lake is huge and would take a lifetime to walk around it, there are some pleasant walks within sight of the city centre which I took advantage of. The trade show was held over a four day period and by the end of it I was tired but pleased to have been able to attend, it brought about a degree of normality into my life.

The following Sunday, we were invited to take our friends to a narrow boat rally at Rickmansworth, by the owners of *Arcturus* and *Sirius*, which were my grandparents' boats.

Whilst there I also had the chance to meet up with a long lost relative, now in her eighties, that I hadn't met before. Helen was my grandfather's niece, making her my second cousin and was connected to the canal boat scene through her father, Tommy Woodhouse who was married to my grandfather's sister and was also a captain of another narrow boat, *Electra* which was also moored and on display at Rickmansworth and owned by the son of the man who owns *Arcturus*. It was quite a nostalgic day and one I would not have missed for the world.

Thursday 3rd June 1999

Appointment to see my specialist, Dr Roques in his clinic. Blood count is satisfactory and collected more drugs from pharmacy department. Due to go into day ward the following Monday for more Pamidronate to strengthen my spine. Followed by much of the same due on Friday 2nd July.

With all hospital appointments out of the way and the doctors saying that I was fit enough to travel a little further afield, we departed on the previously arranged holiday to Lake Maggiore, one of the northern Italian lakes by coach with our friends. It is a little tiring having to go overland, but as our friends and travelling companions don't fly, it's our only opportunity of being able to enjoy going away on holiday with them. There are compensations however in travelling with an organised group in so much as there would always be someone on hand to carry suitcases and take them up to the hotel bedroom. We were due to be away from Saturday 3rd July until Sunday 11th 1999, and we fully intended to make up for last year's cancelled holiday through the onset of my disease. As with most coach journeys to the continent, it involved the coach trip from our local pick up point to Dover docks, before boarding a cross channel ferry at tea-time. The short passage to Calais is under an hour and a half, from where the coach drove us to our first overnight hotel stop on the outskirts of Paris. The Radisson SAS hotel at Charles De Gaulle airport is a splendid modern hotel with every conceivable facility. I could have happily spent three or four days there watching the aeroplanes and the rabbits burrowing under the runway. The motorway into Paris also goes underneath the runway at some point and it will be interesting to see how many years it takes the rabbits to completely undermine the runway causing it to collapse onto the road bringing the whole of Paris to a standstill from both the air and the road.

After an enforced detour around the Grand Saint Bernard pass because the tunnel was closed following the disastrous fire, we made a pit stop at a Mövenpick restaurant at Martigny. This establishment put all English motorway service stations to absolute shame. In addition to a wonderful array of fresh food, pastries and any combination of smoothies you could ever have wished for, there is a verandah over a lake filled with trout, windsurfers and people swimming. The adjacent caravan site and holiday complex was a throng of happy holiday makers, or people like me who having travelled all this way, didn't see the point in going any further into France as this place had the lot! Sadly however, the coach driver rounded us all up again for our final thrash into Italy. I could have very happily stayed there at the Mövenpick for a week or two, but it was ordained that we couldn't and reluctantly boarded the coach. Once on the road again, we were able to look forward to arriving in Italy, and without a doubt, Lake Maggiore is a beautiful place to visit and has three distinctly different islands, known as the Borromean Islands, after Charles Borromeo who was once the overlord of this wonderful area in the Lombardy region of Italy which has been popular with English tourists ever since the Victorians discovered them during the time of the Grand Tours of Europe. The whole area is a delight.

As our friends still had some summer holiday entitlement due to them, and as I was still feeling quite well despite the arduous over land journey, we all headed off on the Wednesday following our trip to Italy, down to Gloucester for a few days. We stayed at the County Hotel in the centre of town just a short walk from the docks and Waterways Museum, which we visited on the Thursday of that week. I found the cine film clip of my grandparents on their canal narrow boats, *Arcturus* and *Sirius* being shown. My sister who had visited the museum earlier arranged for posterity, copies of the film to be made so that we could each have one. Our day also included a trip along the River Severn and a visit to the Museum of Packaging, it sounds an anorakish thing to do, but was actually quite interesting. The usual cries of "I remember those" or "Gracious me, I'd forgotten all about those" could be heard at every exhibit, uttered by both our party and everyone else who stopped to gaze. One man's junk is another man's meal ticket! We returned home on Saturday of that week which was the 30th anniversary of man's walk on the moon.

Friday 23rd July 1999

Worthing Hospital needs to check up on my bone marrow. I have a biopsy under sedation. I am due to have more bone strengthening agent too. Collecting more drugs from pharmacy. Advised of trip to Hammersmith for routine check on 3rd August.

Tuesday 3rd August 1999

Hospital car due at 11:00 for 14:00 appointment. Blood tests conducted. I still feel very good and can cope with most things at present.

The report from Hammersmith Hospital was good, I was making the progress that had been hoped for which was encouraging. My sailing buddy, Alan, has got shingles now, but as I had an injection when Julie's mother became unwell with the virus, I was all right and could go sailing without too much fear of catching the Herpes Zosta infection. Another friend, knowing I was not getting out and about too often, invited me to join him in a trip down to see a colleague in Wiltshire. It was a long tiring day, but as I'd told all my friends, it was my intention to travel around as much as possible whilst I was in remission and I had achieved what I set out to do, even if it did make me very tired.

Julie and myself were also invited to the 25th wedding anniversary of a former work colleague and his wife with whom I had also worked. It was a warm summer's evening so we were able to sit outside for some of the time. A buffet had been laid on and there were many people I knew there, including a number of business acquaintances and friends, I enjoyed their company very much and some even said they were concerned about me, however it was only our close friends who kept in touch. It's an old saying but very true, 'You find out who your friends are in time of crisis' the majority of the people there have not made contact and would have been embarrassed by their inability to say 'the right thing'. By 22:30 that evening I was getting exceptionally tired and we made our apologies and left them all to it in order that I could retire to my bed.

Thursday 9th September 1999

After feeling unwell during the previous day and night, phoned Dr Roques to tell him my temperature was 37.8° Had an appointment with him at 12:00 and he advised I must stay in hospital. Being put into cubicle 9. I had been well for so long and it necessitated me attending the day ward in Worthing for routine infusions of Pamidronate on that Thursday, therefore it came as a bit of a surprise to be told that I've got to be admitted to hospital for an indeterminate period of time, whilst they sorted out my immediate health issue. The next day, Friday the 10th, was my 55th birthday. It wasn't the first time I'd been absent without leave from birthdays and anniversaries, but it certainly wouldn't be the last!

Friday 10th September 1999

My birthday, I'm still feeling very rough and have got a high temperature. Hooked up to saline, oxygen and nebuliser to assist my breathing.

I had many visitors that day, people probably feeling sorry for me having to spend my birthday in hospital, it's something you get used to. Our daughter, Emma brought in a splendidly decorated and iced Marks & Spencer birthday cake, it was taken away by my friends the nurses to be cut up into small pieces. I had one small piece and the nurses enjoyed the rest of it, they don't get fed at home!

Saturday 11th September 1999

Going to take a sleeping pill to help me through the night as feeling very rough. Can't stop shivering, asked for tea with whisky and was most surprised to get it! Told I've got Pneumonia, not good news as it can cause complications. Being put on strong antibiotics.

Sunday 12th September 1999

Still feeling quite poorly and can't stop shivering, temperature around 38°. No sign of going home yet for a few days.

Tuesday 14th September 1999

Told I can go home later today after my drugs have been prepared, can't wait! Finally got out at 14:30.

I should have been down at Poole for a sailing trip that coming weekend with my sailing buddy Alan, it can wait, the sea will still be there ready for me when I'm able to enjoy it. The Chinese take-away would still be there as would be the snooker hall, the proprietor of which only saw us once a year but regarded us a regulars, probably because we took so long to sink the balls during our epic 'best of three' matches that he thought we were part of the furniture. During the next few weeks, life returned to 'normal' with friends and family visiting to enquire as to my well being and I saw Dr Roques in his clinic in Worthing. It was always comforting to learn that all was well and that I was not due up at Hammersmith hospital again until the end of October.

Monday 25th October 1999

Hospital car service due at 08:45 ready for 11:00 appointment at Hammersmith. Due for blood tests and sperm count as my ability to father any more children was almost certainly affected by chemotherapy, not that we wanted another one anyway. A subsequent letter from Jane Apperley confirmed a nil sperm count. It's now approximately a year since my bone marrow transplant and having stayed out of serious trouble, we decided to celebrate my remission by going to Paris for a few days. We drove to Ashford, staying overnight in a Travelodge before catching the 09:30 Eurostar service to Paris Gare du Nord station arriving there in just two hours. The whole journey was so easy and without any fuss or drama. We bought a three day Metro pass which paid for itself twice over and used it to make our way to and from our hotel, the Brebant on Boulevard Poissonnière in the 9th Arrondissement, the Metro station of Grandes Boulevard was immediately outside which made travel very easy indeed. The only exception was that the Metro station had four entrances and exits and special attention had to be paid to which one we used to save us a walk in the snow and rain of 100 yards on the opposite side of the street, but we eventually got it worked out by the time we had to return home!

It was a pity that the weather was so cold, it chilled us to the marrow and much of our time was spent taking coffee and meals in the excellent department stores such as; Galleries Lafaytte and Samaritaine. They were stocked to the hilt with Christmas goods and were decorated magnificently. We ventured up to the second stage of La Tour de Eiffel, the top section being closed as a mist had set in making visibility impossible. The all glass enclosed Bateau Mouche provided both shelter from the cold and a scenic journey down the Seine, we enjoyed both elements. The weather was beginning to affect me and I was quite pleased to be on the 17:15 Eurostar on the next day, Tuesday 23rd for our journey home. We enjoyed our celebratory trip to Paris, but would probably chose to re-visit in the Spring-time, not Winter again. I managed to keep out of trouble and hospital right over the Christmas period, I certainly felt much better this year as compared with last

Christmas. However, I knew it couldn't last and following a visit to the day ward, the inevitable happened.

Wednesday 29th December 1999

Attending day ward in Worthing Hospital for routine blood checks. Told them of some phlegm on my chest. Was told to go home and pack a bag, I was to be admitted and placed on a saline drip and to be given strong antibiotics. It seems quite a common occurrence, missing family events for today is our daughter Emma's birthday. I was in hospital for mine, so why shouldn't I be in for hers?

Friday New Year's Eve 1999

Being sent home today on New Year's Eve with anti-biotic for phlegm (Levofloxacin). Discharged at 15:00.

It was not only New Year's Eve but a dawning of a new century, I stayed up to watch on television the spectacle as it unfolded of a New Year and Millennium around the world. One of the most outstanding light shows was that of Paris and the Eiffel Tower illuminated to represent a rocket taking off, it made me very emotional, as in fact I've been ever since my treatment has begun. I could never watch Lassie Comes Home or Ring of Bright Water at the best of times, now it's impossible for me to watch anything with the slightest degree of emotion in it before I well up and have to excuse myself from the room.

Tuesday 11/01/2000

Due at Worthing hospital for a further bone marrow biopsy to check my progress. Still not quite a 100% from chest infection, don't want to end up with pneumonia again.

Monday 17th January 2000

Due at Hammersmith Hospital again for routine check up, hope they are aware of the results of my recent bone marrow biopsy. Car came 09:15 and we are due home at 16:00 hrs. May be having to have course if Immuglobulin to boost bloods.

Monday 24th January 2000

Having to have x-ray at Worthing Hospital regarding my chest infection.

Wednesday 2nd February 2000

Seeing Dr Roques for medication as tummy upset from all the drugs I'm taking, so he prescribes a new one to me, Metronidazole which promptly makes me very sick indeed. Not due in day ward for another month to have more bone strengthening (Pamidronate).

Monday 10th April 2000

Another routine hospital appointment at Hammersmith, have managed to stay out of trouble for several months now, hope it keeps up. Hospital car came at 09:00 at got to hospital at 10:45, told everything ok and need not go for another six months.

With the news that I was alright and didn't need to report into any hospital for a while, we take another holiday whilst the going is good and following my own philosophies of "If you feel you can travel, then travel and enjoy it", and "Life's too short to only drink the house wine" We drove up to Heathrow and stayed the night in the Novotel hotel close to the airport. It was very civilised and restful, it set us in the right frame of mind for the flight to Milan the next day and on to Lake Como. There was a shuttle bus that called at all the London Heathrow hotels and dropped us at our selected terminal, it was very convenient and saved having to arrange long term car parking at the airport as the hotel had a secure car park at no extra cost to the guests. One of my first rules of air travel, was to book into the private lounges, they were worth every penny and provide the traveller with rest & resuscitation and is far more sensible for someone like me, who must always be vigilant about mixing with people who might cough over me and spread diseases, colds and such like which invariably leads to me being hospitalised with pneumonia which must be avoided at all costs. I appreciated that we were flying and would be in a confined area with recirculated air, but that was a chance we had to take. The benefits of being able to get away on holiday, out weighed the risk of breathing in recycled air for ninety minutes. On arrival at the comparatively new Malpensa airport in Milan, we boarded our coach for the 90 minutes transfer to Menaggio on the shores of Lake Como and followed the road through villages whose houses and villas were bedecked in both white and purple wisteria and looking their best in the late April sun. We arrived at the Grand Hotel Menaggio and immediately bumped into, either the notorious woman murderer, Dr Harold Shipman, or someone who is a dead ringer for him. Do we phone the News of the World or just pretend he doesn't exist? We decided to see if any of the female guests in the hotel went missing mysteriously, and then make a phone call to London.

A quick head count revealed that there was no necessity to be alarmed and we wondered how many other people were playing the "I recognise you as Lobby Ludd and claim my ten shillings" game. For those of you who don't remember such exciting summer seaside holiday events put on by a well known tabloid newspaper in England, ask your mum!

Lake Como is another of the picturesque northern Italian lakes in the Lombardy Region, and like the others, offers outstanding scenery and crisp air as the lakes were formed by the melting snows and glacial waters from the mountains behind them. Queen Victoria and other heads of state enjoyed this region and it was my intention to do similarly, I just had to stay well enough.

Some of the towns and villages that we visited around the immediate area are very attractive, the town of Como itself sits at the southern end of the 'Y' shaped 30-mile lake. There is a magnificent cathedral which we only viewed externally and attractive gardens which lead down to the lakeside where there are many good cafés by the wide piazza overlooking the lake which we took advantage of. Around half a mile from old Como town is the hill top town of Brunate, which is reached by the 100-year-old funicular railway which provided us with a pleasant and memorable excursion, the viewing terrace has a magnificent view over both the town and lake, we thought that we were at the back of beyond until you get up there and see that it's served by a bus route and has a bank serving the thriving business community. For an even better view of the wonderful lake, visitors can take a float plane flight from Como's officially recognized Air Station of the 1930's era, although no buildings exist. Passengers board the plane from a launch. To see how it looked in it's heyday, McDonald's in Como have an art-deco poster of the service upstairs in their restaurant. Nearby is the small lakeside town of Cernobbio, 10km from Como which has a 5-star hotel that charges €1,000 a night for a suite. The Villa D'Este, along with the Hotel Cippriani in Venice, are regarded as two of Italy's finest, we were escorted around the hotel but were offered no hospitality at all, we were too poor! The town of Menaggio, on the Western side of Lake Como, is at its best in early May with wisteria flowering in profusion from the numerous balconies, roof gardens and terraces. The lakeside town is served by both passenger and car ferries which run from the ferry port adjacent to the Grand Hotel Menaggio which has a Four Star plus rating. The views from the dining room across the lake are magnificent. The hotel has an outdoor swimming pool, but very few were brave enough to venture into it during our April stay at the hotel where we were treated as guests, rather than part of a packaged tour and put into inferior rooms or had to eat in a separate dining room which occurs so often when travelling with an organized tour from the major operators, no names mentioned but most of the passengers are known as 'Wallies'. Our dining room at the Grand Hotel Menaggio was a bright and airy room, which could be, and was opened up to catch the morning sun rising from behind the mountain to flood the room with warmth and sunlight. The head waiter was a very professional man from the town of Stresa on Lake Maggiore, he was delighted to know that we thought very highly of his home town, having stayed in a hotel there the year before. Menaggio is a prosperous town and once had a railway link to Como itself. The erstwhile station adjacent to our hotel is now a supermarket selling everything from dogs' beds to doughnuts. Many locals and visitors alike would like to see the railway line reinstated as the two other forms of transport are either laboriously slow on the ferry service, which doesn't matter if you're on holiday, or at the mercy of the single carriageway road which gets very congested and takes just one accident to entirely close the road for hours. Since there is no alternative road to take, you just have to sit it out. The ferry service is a wonderfully organized facility and provides water transport by passenger ferry, car ferry or the high speed Hydrofoil which is ideal for getting about if you are in a hurry. However, it's twice the price of the conventional ferry service and on hot days you are enclosed in the cabin and miss the benefit of a cooling breeze whilst plying the lake. At least there is a choice, which you don't get on the road. The nearby town of Tremezzo, has the most famous and imposing of all the lakeside villas, Villa Carlotta. Built in 1690 and owned by the Crown Prince of Saxe Meiningen and his wife, Charlotte, after whom the villa was named. The manicured grounds extend to about 14 acres. Springtime is undoubtedly the best season to visit, as we did, it was wonderful as the shrubs are in full bloom. The most convenient way of visiting Villa Carlotta is by ferry boat, as the service from Como town stops immediately outside the main entrance. A short walk from Villa Carlotta is the moored up and retired paddle steamer *Bisbino* now converted into a café and restaurant in which we enjoyed a pleasant meal and drink. A full account of its restoration and conversion is portrayed in photographs in the main saloon where jazz evenings are held in the summer.

From Menaggio town, runs a regular bus service which we take along with other guests who have perceived that it's a lot cheaper than going on the organized tour from the hotel, passes close to the local hospital (we make a note of that in case it's ever needed) through the Swiss border to the town of Lugano which stands on the lake of the same name. The town is vibrant and has an obviously wealthy air about it. The numerous jewellery shops display precious metals and diamonds, but not their prices. If you need to ask the price, you can't afford it. Boutiques have designer clothes and large price tags, this is a town for the seriously rich shopper which we're not. A worthwhile excursion, is to take another ferry boat ride from Lugano town, to the small and delightful village of Gandria and explore the narrow winding streets. The houses and restaurants are all crammed into an impossibly small area and cling to the steep terraces, it's a wonderful place to visit and we would happily return on every perceivable occasion. Lugano is easily reached by rail and road thanks to the longest motorway tunnel in the world, the Saint Gottard, which is nearly 17 km long and has an accompanying railway line. Once described as the Rio de Janeiro of the continent, but I didn't hear anyone describe it as such whilst I was there, everyone did say however, how beautiful the area was and a return visit was more than just a possibility.

I had managed yet again to survive the trip without need to report into a hospital or doctor's surgery and felt pleased for myself and my wife Julie who would have the added responsibility of looking after my well being and administering additional medication. The missed sailing trip to Poole was reorganised for the week-end of 12th May. My sailing buddy collected me en-route to Poole, where we reached our rented mobile home by 15:00, just enough time for a sail if we could organize ourselves, which we did. By tradition, our sailing weekends also include three games of snooker and a huge Chinese take-away. Our standard of play doesn't improve as we only ever play once a year, and that's always against each other, we take it in turns to win.

Chapter Four.

Still in remission, still travelling.

It was now almost exactly two years since my Multiple Myeloma was diagnosed in May 1998 and eighteen months since the bone marrow transplant was conducted at Hammersmith Hospital. With an 'average' period of remission being thirty months, or so we were told, I have at least a year in hand to travel. Every opportunity has to be taken no matter whether it's trips within England, the Continent or further afield.

I still had the wanderlust and the ability to get around, so with our travelling companions, we head off to the pretty East Sussex harbour town of Rye, just an hour and a half from our home town. We were booked into Jeakes House which was situated up the cobbled and beautiful, Mermaid Street amongst the other picturesque and historic houses in this delightful town. The Ship Inn close to the harbour had whitebait on their lunch menu, I could never refuse these little fishes and saw no reason to do so on this occasion. In fact three of us decided that the offer was too good to refuse and, as usual, we enjoyed them throughout the whole of the afternoon.

The town of Rye is one of the ancient Cinque Ports with a castle fortification to keep the marauding French from reaching the town up the River Rother on which it stands. Some French soldiers succeeded and were imprisoned in Ypres Tower, now a museum. It's worth the climb to the top of the church tower to take in the surrounding countryside and distant views to the sea. We found a tea shop and then retired to the hotel for a rest before venturing out to find a restaurant for our evening meal. The outside of one of the restaurants looked promising and if the accolades were to be believed, would suit us admirably. Owned and run by Mr Medallion Man who's wife was in sole charge of operating the microwave to reheat, and ruin, the already prepared meals by their gourmet chef (if the accreditation is to be believed). The owner's large dog did very well for himself on the leftovers, of which there were plenty, never again will we revisit Medallion Man. Beware when reading menus in other towns when it says "Medallions of Lamb" the restaurant might just be run by one of his relatives! The following day we drove to another hopelessly pretty village, Winchelsea which was rebuilt by Edward I after the original village was submerged in the 13th century by sea erosion. The town is now laid out in formal fashion around a village green and is widely believed to be the first attempt at town planning. There was an art exhibition being held in the 14th century Court Hall which also has a small jail where the prisoners, probably French as they invaded three times, were held prior to their hearing in the court and being transported to the Ypres Tower in neighbouring Rye.

For our last night dinner, we visited the pre-booked Old Forge Restaurant in Rye, which from the outside and its geographical location, does not look inspiring. However, the meal was cooked to order in the open plan kitchen so the diners could see the whole cooking process, chef would present the uncooked steak or fish to you for approval before cooking it to your specific liking. We would gladly re-visit the Old Forge Restaurant the next time we were in Rye. A huge bowl of Moules in a clear stock followed by a thick fillet steak, cooked to perfection. We returned home on Saturday 20th May in time for me to have a short rest and start packing in preparation of me flying to Geneva on the Monday to accompany my friend in the meetings industry, David. When we collected our luggage in Geneva, it was apparent that British Airways had decided to use my suitcase as a wheel chock for the aeroplane and David's luggage must have held some total fascination for the baggage handlers, as they had managed to open it and let it travel round the carousel with the contents in full view of the other passengers.

It cost BA two new suitcases at exorbitant prices from a plush city centre luggage store. Before flying home on the Friday, I took myself off on a lake cruise on one of the splendid old steamers that ply Lake Geneva. So soporific was the movement through the water, that I fell asleep and missed half of the journey. Still it probably did me a lot of good. I got home at 21:00 that evening, tired but glad I made the trip, I love Geneva and will try to go again next year if I'm deemed well enough.

Monday 5th June 2000

Due at Worthing Hospital for bone strengthening infusion in morning and local G.P.'s for a Tetanus injection in the afternoon. Seems ages ago since last at hospital. Still feeling quite well, not much pain, being kept under control by taking Dihydrocodine tablets.

Monday 19th June 2000

Due at dentists in Rustington for x-ray, scale and polish. All preventative treatment, just in case any mouth ulcers develop and cause problems in the future.

I'd been let out of the house again, another trip down to Rockley Point, Poole with my sailing buddy, Alan. Usual routine of; sailing, a swim (if French girls were in the Jacuzzi), snooker, which neither of us play at any other time during the year, a Chinese take-away, a few beers and sink into our respective beds. We always treat ourselves to a cooked breakfast from Alberto's on the quay because it might be the only time we get to eat until the evening, and it's quite amusing to order a full vegetarian breakfast with sausage and bacon from an Italian restaurant at 07:00. A note of interest here, I've got wet suits older than most of the waitresses!

We used to frequent a café next door to the fishing tackle shop, until the owner sold up and the new proprietors put lace doilies on the new round pine tables and made it clear that lug-worms and toast should be kept apart as far as possible. Suitably re-fuelled and depending upon how cold and wet it was outside once we had our already damp wet-suits on, a last cup of coffee with a slug of Southern Comfort in it. We would then rig the boat and get out on the water for a full days sailing. The café close to the ferry at Sandbanks had recently been redecorated prior to the commencement of the new tourist season. It just goes to show how churlish some people can be, we arrived in pouring rain on the beach adjacent to the café, rain water dripping off our sailing suits and in desperate need of a cup of coffee. . . He wouldn't let us in, we had to sit in the continuing rain on his terrace with diluted coffee and soggy doughnuts! Just to restore your faith in human nature, Alan booked a morning's session for us on a brand new Hobie Cat 18 foot catamaran, as a treat. We got out into open water and the wind died to practically nothing, not quite the invigorating sail we had hoped for. On our return to the beach, the owner of the Cat centre didn't charge us as we hadn't had a decent sail, decent of him or what?

Another holiday jaunt started today, Monday 3rd July, this time to visit another of the Italian lakes, Lake Garda. We haven't been before although our travelling companions, Bill and Barbara have. I feel quite well and our American Express travel insurance is fully comprehensive and paid for, so we have no hesitation in setting forth again. After the familiar journey to Dover docks and ferry to Calais, we travel by coach to Dunkerque for an over night stop before heading down through France en route to our second night stop at the delightful Alsace town of Offenburgh where there are some very tactile bronze sculptures. Just like the bust of Juliet in

Verona, the breast areas of the statues were shiny in comparison to the rest of the figure! The next morning, after a substantial breakfast of cold meat and cheeses, we head off towards Italy and pass through Hornberg in the Black Forest.

The small village must be the Cuckoo Clock capital of the world for there were more shops selling them than any other town. It also boasted the largest clock in the world, which is the size of a small cottage with a real chimney that smokes and on the hour a full size sweep emerged covered in soot, whilst the shop owner passes round glasses of Cherry Brandy, which was watered down. It was still only 09:00 in the morning. If you were tempted into his shop which has a thousand clocks all ticking away and chiming at different intervals, you get a glass full of the real and very potent liqueur. We pressed on without purchasing a cuckoo clock or succumbing to Cherry Brandy. This was our second day of coach travel and I was getting bored with the constant stops made by the coach driver every hour and a half, it took for ever to get down to Italy! The driver, at the commencement of the journey, announced that the coach has tea and coffee making facilities on board and for the price of a strip of cloakroom tickets, we can redeem them for a drink. It is therefore in his interest that he says every 90 minutes, "I expect you'd like to stop for a cup of tea wouldn't you?" To which our fellow travellers, most of whom are octogenarians, say, "Yes please!" We reached Torbole on Lake Garda on our third day of coach travel and tea drinking. A snap shot impression of the lake and surrounding area follows;

Torbole, Lake Garda.

A small lake side town of just 2,500 permanent residents which is swelled tenfold during the summer months by the arrival of the tourists, of which we make up a small percentage. This lake is yet another in the Lombardy region of Italy and the area takes its name from an invading tribe of barbarians in the 6th Century, the Lombards. Today it is us who are invading this delightful spot. Ferry boats ply the length and breadth of the lake which is a sailor's paradise and at any one time dozens of small craft vie with the ferries for access to harbour entrances. Torbole is situated near the northern end of the lake, close to Riva del Garda which is the largest of the towns and is its commercial centre. All walks of human life promenade along the vibrant lakeside pathways with copious quantities of seats provided to allow careful study and observation of the flora, fauna and local residents who make up this colourful montage of images. An elderly man walks past with a young bird on his arm, "Don't touch her, she mine all mine!" he exclaims to all who approach, "These parrots can give a nasty bite!" We continue our walk stopping for refreshment at every opportunity, soaking up the sun and the culture. To the rear of the town is an ancient mule track that leads through olive groves and along cobbled stoned paths as it snakes its way up to the hillside hamlet of Nago. It gives the impression of being miles away from civilisation, a fact endorsed by a ruined castle on one of the hills and general lack of activity about the place. We learn however that just beyond the village is a bus route which uses the main road into Torbole past a local landmark in the shape of a rock formation, called The Giant's Kettle, or Gigante Marmite. At least we took the pretty route.

A short ferry ride away is the town of Malcesine with a small bustling harbour around which are brightly painted houses and cafés. To the rear of the town, up a steep flight of wide steps is the cable car to Monte Baldo, which we take and enjoy the spectacular views from the summit and our picnic, bought from the supermarket in the town prior to boarding the ride. There are magnificent views across the town to the lake with the ferry boats chugging back and forth to Torbole and Riva. I returned to Torbole in a taxi after an unexpected interlude in hospital.

Sunday 9th July 2000

Feeling unwell at Malcesine, shivering a lot and drinking coffee to try and warm up. Our friends go off and buy a thermometer and establish my temperature is 39° The café owner calls an ambulance and I'm taken to the local hospital. My condition is explained and drugs given to bring my temperature down are administered. I stay there for three hours before being put into a taxi and driven back to the hotel.

Monday 10th July 2000

The doctor was called and a prescription given to the porter who returned with drugs within forty minutes. I still had a temperature and had to stay indoors until it had stabilised. Put on a fruit and yoghurt diet and told to drink lots of water. American Express were contacted, who said I must stay in Torbole until completely better and then they would fly me home.

What a result! Our friends departed within the next few days by coach for their three day overland journey and we transferred to the hotel owner's sister hotel just to the rear of the town where a room was made available to us for as long as we needed. The drugs did their job, the fever subsided and my digestion returned to normal. We could now enjoy what was left of our holiday. Feeling so much better and able to resume our travels, we board the ferry to the small village of Limone on the western shore of the lake. It's so pretty there with lemon trees growing around the small harbour, the waterside cafés and restaurants. It is one of the most delightful places we have visited and would go back if possible. We take a last look at Riva, missing the ferry and hailing a taxi for the short trip back to Torbole.

One the most well known towns on Lake Garda is Sirmione with its castellated walls and unique position of being on a promontory at the southern end of the lake which is considerably wider than the northern end at Riva. Michael Schumacher has a house here. There are many other delightful towns to visit, but not this time sadly, we shall have to return to finish our sight seeing.

Friday 14th July 2000

The private ambulance car, come mini coach arrives at 08:30 and drives us to Verona Airport where we are put into an executive lounge awaiting our boarding on the BA flight at 12:00 for Gatwick. Put in Club Class and fed Lobster and chicken for lunch, good job I feel so much better so as to enjoy it.

On arrival at Gatwick, we were met by a chauffeur and driven to our front door. I shall always recommend American Express as a travel insurance provider and urge any traveller not to set foot outside their front door unless they have insurance cover. We spoke to our friends who had also just arrived home after a horrendous three day journey with people being ill and one lady taken to hospital in France and left there as she was too ill to travel any further. It could easily have been me, had it not been for the fact that we announced to the insurers immediately, that a problem was about to manifest itself.

Thursday 20th July 2000

Seeing Dr Roques in his clinic in Worthing following my set back in Italy. He prescribed even more drugs but, otherwise says I'm OK.

Monday 14th August 2000

Due at day ward for usual infusion of Pamidronate, feeling quite OK. Next one due on 08/09/2000 as we will be away in four weeks time to Essex. I manage to stay out of hospital this year on my birthday and head off up to Great Dunmow in Essex, close to Stansted Airport to see my nephew. We travelled home on the 13th September without any medical emergencies.

Monday 25th September 2000

Being collected by hospital car service at 08:45 as due to see Dr Apperley at Hammersmith hospital. Blood samples were taken and all is still right. I'm now in that situation of not needing to be seen more frequently than six months, but anything could start to happen again within the next few months.

If Hammersmith said that I'm all right, then I was all right to travel again, accordingly, we flew out to Seville from Gatwick today, the 28th September. As per my previous rules of flying, we were booked into a private lounge and enjoyed the facilities before joining our flight at 17:50 arriving at our hotel, the Inglaterre at 21:45. It was a nice hotel in a good location close to the town centre and overlooking a square. For those who have yet to visit Seville, a short description follows;

Seville has a population of some 700,000 inhabitants, with a very diverse heritage and ethnic background. What is absolutely apparent to the first time visitor is that all who live there have a deep routed sense of belonging, not just to their city, but to the region of Andalucia and Spain itself. Steeped in history, this is Spain's second largest city. It was once occupied by the Carthaginians in the year 500 BC, who called the city, Hispalis. Later the Romans came, under Julius Caesar who promptly renamed it Julia Romula, or Little Rome. The emperor 'Trojan' gave his name to the river which runs through the city, and to the north bank, both of which became known as Triana.

Seville is reputed to be the home and origin of Flamenco dancing, practised by the Andalucian women who were descended from the slaves imported from Cadiz to the south west. The city also produced the distinctive glazed tiles, known as Azulejo which have a golden appearance and adorn the roof of the city's Torre del Oro, or Golden Tower. It is a twelve-sided tower built by the Moors in 1220 on the bank of the river now known as the Guadalquivier, or Big River. The tower stands just as resplendent today as it did hundreds of years ago and is now used as a maritime museum with an indigenous date palm standing beside it which says much for the climate here. Numerous orange trees and a banana plant of some considerable proportion can be seen within the grounds of the university. The enormous building was formerly the state tobacco factory and its history is inexorably linked with Bizet's Carmen, where girls like her would roll the tobacco leaves on their thighs to make cigars. Bizet captured the essence of a dusky maiden enslaved into a work-house and immortalized her forever in his opera of the same name. The other link that Seville has to opera, is that it was used as the setting for Mozart's Marriage of Figaro. Near to the university, is the splendidly ornate and exotic Alphonso XIV hotel with Moorish architecture and an enclosed courtyard into which non-residents are allowed access and marvel at the fine carvings and other artefacts of the period. The city is a working port, although there is little evidence of shipping activities today. Still standing on the river bank is a hand operated crane for unloading the cargoes from the ships' holds. It took a team of four men to operate it. The port made Seville one of the richest cities in the world, renowned for being the only Spanish city allowed to trade with America between 1503 and 1680. During that time, cargoes of silk and tobacco made considerable fortunes for the merchants and spending on a grand scale was undertaken to show off the city's wealth. Many of the opulent buildings still adorn the streets, although most have been taken over by the city for offices and administration centres. There was also a railway track and steam engine to transport the unloaded cargoes from the port to the railway station, sadly neither are still there. The station is now a shopping mall although its wonderful Moorish façade still remains. Known now as 'Les Plaza des Armas', the shopping centre has numerous food outlets, boutiques and a supermarket. The permanent way in front of the former station has been removed which is now an impressively large piazza with a modern hotel built adjacent to it. Rail passengers now have a new station at San Justa on the outskirts of the city in the direction of the modernised airport. The new high speed trains connect Seville with Madrid and Barcelona. However a journey to Barcelona, city centre to city centre, takes five hours on the train and only two hours on the bus!

Seville boasts the largest Gothic building in the world in its cathedral, La Magna Hispalensis. Built between 1172 and 1195 by the Almohads, it stands on a site of a former mosque erected 50 years prior to Christianity. The tower was retained and its height increased to 319 feet to match the overall scale and grandeur of the building. It has a huge weather vane named 'Faith', or 'Giralda' and the tower is now known as the Giralda Tower which is visible from most parts of the city and acts as a landmark for visitors who have lost their direction whilst traversing the myriad of narrow streets and alleyways that make up the city's Barrio quarter. The tower is an exact replica of the Koutoubia in Marrakech, Morocco also built under the Almohads first leader, Abdelmoumen. The cathedral, which is the second largest church after the Basilica in Rome, contains the tomb and letters of the explorer Christopher Columbus brought from Havana in 1899 after Cuba became an independent country. There are strong ties between the two countries, because of their cigar manufacturing industry. The district behind the cathedral, is the former Jewish community of Santa Cruz, known locally as 'The Barrio'. Its inhabitants can be seen giving impromptu performances of the Flamenco dance. No excuse to dance is needed and their musical accompaniment can be nothing more than a piece of corrugated cardboard strummed to destruction by the deft fingers of a foot tapping musician of the most basic genre. Seville is a vibrant city and has three distinct development periods. Firstly there is the old part whose cultures and architecture date from the 12th century, followed by the Iberia-America Exposition of 1929 which saw the construction of decorative pavilions as trade centres. The exposition occupied a vast area of the city, now known as the Marie Luisa Park after a previous Queen of Spain.

The third and most recent development, and possibly the most unsuccessful, was the 1992 World Fair which although it attracted some 40 million visitors, cost the city eight billion pesetas to construct, from which it has never really recovered the cost involved. The new railway and station was built, the airport enlarged and modernised, the river was diverted and canalised to make it less prone to flooding. The area on which the site stands is at the opposite end of the city to the exposition of 1929, which it tried to emulate. The lack of funds in the city's coffers is reflected in the present condition of the site, known as la Cartuja. Much of the area is in decline and only the 50 metre Banesto tower is in use as a communications tower. The site is close to the densely populated tenements of the city and a shanty town, it should never have been built. The site also has two other tall structures, the mock-up of Europe's first space rocket, Arianne and the Tower Mirador which stands infront of the Pavilion of Discovery and acts as an advertisement for a major lift and elevator company. On the river itself is a replica of Ferdinand Magellan's boat, *Victoria* in which he circumnavigated the globe along with several sailors from Seville whose names are immortalised on a bronze and copper monument on the Triana, or north bank of the river. The name Triana emanates from the old Trojan word for river. On the Puerto del Triana, (Bridge of Triana), stands a former watchtower with an ornate clock. The tower is now a fine restaurant with a terrace on its top floor which gives a commanding view over the river and city. The house special is a platter of sea food washed down with copious amounts of ice cold Fino sherry.

End of Travelogue.

Whilst staying at The Inglaterra Hotel in Seville, we happened to meet a most delightful lady, Carol Rilling, resplendently dressed and bearing the sash of the Daughters of the American Revolution, she was a very interesting and enterprising lady of great charm and elegance. Looking resplendent in her "chain of office" as the National Chairman of the Overseas Committee she is a perfect ambassador for this august body of women. Carol has a love of travel and had worked hard to fund a trip to Europe. At that time she was unaware of her ancestors in England and only discovered them much later when she was invited to a meeting of the Daughters of the American Revolution. Eager to become a member, she set about tracing her ancestry. Subsequently, Carol's entitlement to be a member of "the Daughters", emanates from her being the thirteenth descendant of William Mullins of

Dorking, in England's leafy county of Surrey. The building in which he lived is still in existence and a plaque announces the connection of the former occupier to the Pilgrim Fathers. It was here that the Mullin's eldest daughter, Priscilla, was born in 1590 and left Dorking in 1608 along with 90 others, including a group of separatists from Nottingham, to sail in a Dutch ship for a new life in America. The passage was not a direct one as initially they sailed to Amsterdam and a year later to Leiden. The Reverend John Robinson wrote to the town council seeking permission to settle whilst provisioning and recruiting other crew members for their epic voyage. He received a reply on the 12th of February 1609 granting such consent. The provisioning process took considerably longer than anyone had imagined, and they stayed at the port for eight years whilst they were preparing the *Mayflower*, and establishing a crew. The Rev. Robinson and his companions bought a piece of land, called Groene Poort (Green Close) near the Pieterskerk, (St Peter's Church) which later became known as the English Alley. They built 21 small houses, today there stands the Jean Pesijn almshouses, erected in 1683. During that time a diary was maintained by a crew member, William Brewster, an elder of the church who with his adopted son, William Bradford, established The Pilgim Press in 1617. Brewster wrote of the dissatisfaction of the passengers and questioned viability of the voyage as the vessel was deemed to be unseaworthy and returned to England. It was decided that they should not make the passage unescorted and a sister vessel was purchased, the *Speedwell*. Finally, both ships were fully provisioned and sailed from Plymouth, but both boats were proven to be unseaworthy for such an epic voyage and turned back to Plymouth again. By this time a number of the passengers felt that they could no longer face another attempt at the crossing. It had been as long as ten years for some of the crew since the first voyage was embarked upon. Those that remained, set sail in the *Mayflower* and finally landed at Cape Cod in North Virginia on the 26th. November 1620, after a voyage that had lasted for 65 days. Because the colony had become so extended in

Leiden during the time spent there preparing, it was necessary for the Pilgrims to acquire further vessels for the migration. In 1621 the Fortune set sail followed in 1623 by the *Anne* and *Little James*, with a second *Mayflower* leaving in 1629. The first Thanksgiving Day was celebrated in 1621 in honour of the landing. It has endured to this day as one America's most important festivals together with Independence Day on the 4th. of July. The "Boston Tea Party" of 1773 is widely considered to have been the cause of the conflict known as the War of Independence. When the settlers landed they were surprised to hear that many of the native Indians spoke English. They were ancestors of the early settlers, probably fishermen, who along with the Vikings sought out the fish stocks that abounded in the area. Records do not show which of Carol's ancestors (in America) were called to fight in the American Revolution (1776 to 1783), but her research has found another twelve lines of ancestors from England. She has visited the shop in Dorking and the Somerset village of Barton St. David where some of the other ancestors lived.

Friday 6th October2000

Due at Worthing Hospital for bone strengthening infusion. Feeling a bit shivery. Temperature taken at home of 37.9° so went back to hospital and saw Dr. Roques I told him of my intention to fly off to Chicago on Sunday, he advises against it. Had to tell my friend, David, that I couldn't fly with him to Chicago as my doctor forbade it. If I had needed any hospital treatment whilst over there, Amex would check with Dr. Roques and refuse to pay out, I therefore couldn't take the risk of travelling without cover. One day, one day I would manage to get to America, I hadn't achieved it yet, but there was still time, hopefully.

Wednesday 13th December 2000

Not feeling at all well today, temperature is rising. Went to Worthing Hospital at 10:00 for blood tests, told to go home and report back later for results of tests. Went back at 16:30 for a prescription of antibiotic (Amoxylin). No need to be admitted.

Whilst at the hospital, we mentioned to Dr. Roques that we wanted to fly to Madeira for Christmas and was it in order to do so. He insisted that the course of antibiotics be taken and it should give me sufficient cover over the Christmas and New Year holiday. So with the blessing of the good Dr. Roques, we were collected by taxi and driven to Gatwick for the 13:00 flight to Funchal on the so called 'Garden Isle' of Madeira. The weather was disappointing in the first week as it rained intermittently, we hoped for better next week. The island is a popular haunt for English visitors, particularly at this time of year. The gardens are full of exotic plants and yhey grow to enormous size, what we would put in a small flower pot, they have growing wild in monstrous proportions. I continued to take the antibiotics and warded off any further threat of pneumonia. As we hadn't been to Madeira before, the whole island was a new experience to us and we travelled to both the east and west soaking up the culture and the dramatic scenery that the island has to offer. Our hotel was a modern, four star rated, high rise edifice with a shopping mall on the ground and first floors and nine floors of lounges and bedrooms above. The open air swimming pool was above the second floor shopping area, I swam for the first time in two years and felt very pleased with myself. As the town centre was only a mile and a half from the hotel, we often would use the walk as an excuse to stretch our legs. If however, rain threatened during our first week, we would catch the bus which ran very frequently between town and hotel.

The holiday in Madeira did us both a lot of good, we could really relax over the two week period even though we kept ourselves very active with all the sight seeing and walking. I had shaken off all traces of the infection that I took to Madeira and I felt well.

Friday 5th January 2001

The first hospital appointment of the new year, routine visit for Pamidronate. The next clinic appointment is not until 01/02/2001, just routine to ensure that things are still all right, followed by more Pamidronate the day after.

A friend in the financial services industry was holding a seminar in a smart hotel in Croydon and invited me to attend so that I could eat at his expense and drink as much wine as I liked. It was fortuitous that I stuck with coffee as my eldest nephew phoned me on my mobile whilst returning from Croydon to say that he was at Gatwick and needed to be driven to Cambridge. Apparently he had a company medical and they had discovered a potential problem that would require hospitalisation, but he didn't want to be driven there in an ambulance so Julie and myself were called upon to come to his assistance. We stepped in to help and had a few days in Cambridge as a short break away. It was totally unexpected, but quite often those impromptu jaunts are more enjoyable than those planned over a number of weeks. It was not as if he was poorly, his company just wanted it sorted immediately. Whilst up in Cambridgeshire, we all had tea and scones in a delightful tin shack, the Orchard in Grantchester where Rupert Brooke often spent an hour or two writing. His most memorable poem being 'The Old Vicarage, Grantchester' the penultimate lines of which recount,

Stands the church clock at ten-to-three

And is there honey still for tea?

Quite by chance I gazed at the church clock and was amazed that we had timed our visit to co-inside with these revered words, it was 14:50. I didn't however check my own watch, for all I know the clock's hands may have been showing that time for years. But it did add something to the presence of being there. I wanted to send a post card of the tea house to our holiday making friends and on leaving the car park espied a post box and jumped out. As did three photographers hoping to get a scoop photograph of Jeffrey Archer who lived next door and had been in the news for his extramarital activities in the Caribbean. Was I flattered or offended to be mistaken for such a prominent personality? Amused more like, particularly as we all know what ultimate fate befell him. He's got a nice house though, but if it were mine, I'd get the post box moved, or the tea rooms, or the village itself, it wouldn't cost much and I could afford it.

We returned home to West Sussex and left our nephew with the prospect of undergoing an operation to install a pacemaker in the near future. There always seems to be a medical issue somewhere to address in our family. On Friday 23rd January 2001, my daughter and I went to London's Olympia to a Spanish property exhibition. It was a reconnaissance to establish if there was any mileage in forging links with a Spanish developer for Emma to establish herself in my friend's estate agency as a specialist in overseas properties. The idea appealed to her as redundancy from her employer was looming over her. It transpired that many an agency would have been interested, however legislation was changing and all Spanish property sales would have to be conducted from a company with an office in Spain, which we couldn't aspire to. It was a good day out though and we enjoyed ourselves and the hospitality of the various stand holders who would ply us with Sangria and sardinas.

Friday 2nd March 2001

Appointment at Worthing Hospital for Pamidronate, out quite early. Went on from hospital to Donatello's Italian restaurant in Brighton.

The following day we visited our favourite travel agent in a nearby village and booked to fly to Sorrento. I think they were rather surprised when we returned the week after with our daughter to book a week in Spain. We had to settle on a self-catering week in Tenerife.

Monday 12th March 2001

Due up at Hammersmith Hospital for a check-up and an infusion of Haemoglobulin. A fairly uneventful day, spent mostly on the M25 in a traffic queue, or in the hospital's day ward. We arrived home at 16:00 hours quite exhausted but safe in the knowledge that I am still all right.

With our Tenerife holiday coming up shortly. I ordered the currency from our local Post Office and reserved the car parking space at London's Gatwick Airport. With three of us travelling it is cheaper than return rail fares, not that the cost was shared of course, Dad'll pay. Later that day, Emma and myself were due to go to Sandown Park, Esher, Surrey for the Overseas Property exhibition, however we decided against it as the car developed an oil leak. We stayed at home trying to get to grips with the Spanish language tape and phrase book she bought, "Tres moi importante para mi" It is very important for me, to learn something of the language.

We packed our suitcases and all three of us were looking forward to our holiday on Tenerife. We drove up to Gatwick (40 mins), parked and checked in by twelve noon. After a Family Bucket of KFC, we headed for the Servisair lounge and hit the free booze, crisps and nuts. The flight took off at 15:30 and we landed at the newish south terminal in Tenerife at 17:45. The apartment complex in which we were due to stay, the Laguna Park 11, was a modern complex with an unheated sea water pool, it was freezing in there! It had been absolutely years since our family spent a holiday together, and even longer since we had to fend for ourselves! In the days of holidays with the family in our touring caravan, there was little choice, you either catered for yourselves in the caravan, bought fish and chips, or you had to drive home because you couldn't afford to eat out at every mealtime. It was then, with some fear and trepidation, that I agreed to embark upon the "hunter-gatherer" scenario again with a family holiday, fending for ourselves in Tenerife during March 2001. To be honest, it wasn't my first choice for a holiday. I had designs on going to Malta; it would have been new territory and quite different to the volcanic landscape which I saw in Madeira over the previous Christmas, and would see exactly the same again in Tenerife but the travel agent couldn't get us a booking to Malta at relatively short notice, so we had to settle on the Canaries on a self-catering deal. That in itself should have told me something, however, I was too intent in getting away from the chill of English weather, being well enough to travel with my specialist's consent and was seduced by the prospect of sunshine everyday. The accommodation, set in Laguna Park's II complex, was at Torviscas Alto, 1km inland from the waterfront at Puerto Colon should have pre-warned me to the fact that "alto" means high and high means hills. However, I knew that we would cope, as we had built up our leg muscles whilst walking Madeira's hilly terrain. Having arrived at the on-site shop (which purports to be allied to Tesco's) just as it was closing and missed out on our supper, we plundered the uneaten crisps and nuts filched from the Servisair lounge and settled for that. A nightcap in the entertainment lounge, gave us another chance to "snack-out". The apartment comprised; a one double bedroom, a lounge with kitchen at one end, and a bathroom with toilet. We had the bedroom and our daughter the fold-up bed/settee in the lounge. This gave her the opportunity to go out night-clubbing and not disturb us. Having been to the immediate area on three previous occasions, our daughter knew where we could eat and how to get there. A taxi is the most convenient form of transport on the island, and it seems to matter not where you wish to be dropped off, the fare was always 500 Pesetas which is around two pounds.

If we were staying at a hotel, the additional cost of a taxi incurred in going out, and the cost of a dinner, wouldn't exist. So on top of having to take extra money for meals, we had to budget for getting to and from a local resort for dinner. And of course, there was no entertainment in the restaurant, apart from watching the waiters attempting to open a bottle of inferior sparkling wine and making it appear like Moet and Chandon! Therefore, further pesetas were spent on getting another taxi from the restaurant to a large hotel which had a dance floor and "combo" band. As the resorts of Playa las Americas and Los Christianos cater for a strongly Germanic clientele, so too was the style of music played. After a few cocktails, I can slap my (or anybody else's who happens to be nearby) thigh in time with the "beir-keller" melodies with the best of them. A few dark Germanic looks were encountered, as if to say that it is our music and you can't enjoy yourselves also.

Although the entertainment lounge at Laguna Park II did put on a "musical quiz night" and the resident DJ attempted to get the amplifiers to self-destruct by overuse of the bass control, it wasn't for us and we settled into our routine of watching German couples gyrate around a small dance floor in a 5-star hotel and annoy them immeasurably by tapping our feet and slapping our thighs. At least the Germans didn't have to run the gauntlet of the restaurateurs, who line up along the promenade outside their particular establishment, all claiming that "theirs is the best in town and that their wives will kill them, if they don't sell all that she's cooked". After a while, you tend not to look at the menus outside the restaurant, you simply go inside the first one that doesn't have a pushy owner outside. One such establishment was the Aberdeen Steakhouse, a familiar name and from what we saw of the other diners meals, quite acceptable. I don't normally "do" Sangria, but what the heck, when in Rome etc. Subsequently, when our steaks were ordered, we washed them down with copious quantities of the stuff, it is only a fruit cup after all, until you need to get your legs working and then you have this sneaking suspicion that they've spiked it! The restaurant was in the area known as Fänabé, where there are some other self-catering complexes that don't require a route march up the hill before retiring for the night, I must try and remember the area, just in case I ever revisit. Just around the headland from Fänabé, is the Bahia del Duque, or Dukes Bay. On it stands probably the finest hotel on the island, The Gran Hotel Bahia del Duque. To stay at this magnificent hotel, would be a joy beyond belief, but with room prices starting at £300 a night, it is only for the seriously well off. Guests who fall into this category include; Fidel Castro of Cuba, Princess Stephanie of Monaco, Aranxia Sanchez Vicario and Lord Lawrence Olivier's widow, the list is endless. Pre-dinner drinks and cocktail snacks were taken on our balcony at the apartment.

Getting around the island is easy as it has one of the most efficient public transport systems that I have ever encountered, although there are no trains, the bus service puts most other countries to shame. A multi-bay bus station was built ten years ago immediately to the north of Playa de las Americas, at Costa Adeje. Its distinctive green and white buses of the "TITSA" bus line, ply the route up to Santa Cruz every half an hour in perfect comfort in coach-like vehicles. The journey lasts a little over an hour and a quarter, non-stop and takes in some of the dramatic lunar landscape scenery that is typical of the southern half of Tenerife. As the coach approaches Santa Cruz and Puerto de la Cruz in the north, it is obvious that more rain falls here. The small parcels of land are green and residents wear slightly heavier clothing, always a giveaway!

Cruise liners call in at Santa Cruz during their Mediterranean trips, some of the boats I saw there, had been seen earlier on Madeira. There is not much difference between the two islands, especially if you have approached from the sea. There's a town with a harbourside with a backdrop of dramatic tree clad hills, and that's about all! As we were self-catering, I became somewhat of an expert in the cost of meals out. The bus station at Santa Cruz had a wide, polished marble concourse, one part of which was a restaurant. You expect the normal, quick turnover type meals associated with transport cafes, however, a three course meal of soup as a starter, followed by a choice of a pasta dish or chicken "chest" and a sweet, cost around six pounds. Remarkably good value, wholesome and appetising too!

The town of Puerto de la Cruz is slightly smaller than Santa Cruz and has a botanical garden on the top of a hill. The climb is worth every step, just to sample a dish served in the restaurant with a terrace overlooking the town and sea beyond. Their paella is, I maintain, the best there is to be had in the whole of Spain. I should have brought more pesetas with me than I did, although not dear, taking meals out everyday soon erodes into cash reserves. It was therefore fortuitous that on two occasions, the Laguna Park 11 complex, held barbecue evenings. One a Mexican style meal and the other a traditional barbie with an assortment of chicken, steak, bangers and burgers and a jacket potato accompanied by the usual salads etc. All you could eat for six pounds, plus as much local red or white wine, or if you prefer, Sangria. When it comes to drinks, I generally like to see a cocktail of ingredients mixed in front of me, so that I know what's in it. However, this Sangria was pre-mixed and came from a pump, just like lager is served. Having said that, it was probably the best Sangria that I tasted on our holiday, the only thing that detracted from the pleasure, was drinking it out of styrofoam cups, but then hey, so what, it was free!

To sum up our holiday, I don't think that a self-catering arrangement suited us, although I can see that for many families it is ideal and they certainly wouldn't want to be restricted by falling in line with an hotel's regime. As far as value for money is concerned, it wasn't as inexpensive as I thought it would be. Although we were constantly putting our hands into our pockets for meals, whether it be a breakfast to try and "keep us going" through the day, or an evening meal which formed part of our "entertainment", had we used all the facilities provided in the apartment to cater for ourselves, we probably could have saved ourselves some money. This however has to be off set by the fact it was a holiday and not just a trip away from home, a very important issue as far as the "domestic manager" is concerned. A few tips to those on a tight budget would be; to stock up at the local supermarket for breakfast foods, like yoghurts and cereals and eat them "at home". Don't be seduced by the offer of cheap food at a cafe style restaurant on the seafront. They can't afford to give the food away, so they make up their profit by charging a very high price for Cokes and other soft drinks, which all come as a concentrated syrup and cost the restauranteur practically nothing. An example of this practice is; we all walked along the sea front at Playa de las Americas and saw a menu offering sardines, Canarian potatoes and salad for about three pounds, excellent offer we thought. We each had a Coke or Fanta which was served in a balloon shape glass and held almost a litre of drink. Obviously, we were unable to consume it all and priced the same as the meal itself, didn't represent good value for money. This is how they make their profit! I would certainly revisit Tenerife, but next time stay in an hotel. If I am fortunate enough to come up on the Lottery, I will reserve a suite at the Gran Hotel Bahai del Duque. They can charge as much as they wish for drinks, hey, I can afford it! Until then, I just dream. No matter how much eating out cost us, it was still infinitely better than being in Worthing or Hammersmith hospitals eating the luke warm food at no later than half past five in the evening. So being able to get out and about once more was a reward in itself and worth every penny! I just had to stay well enough now and in the future to be able to continue taking those holidays as you just never knew when the opportunity to travel would be denied to you. It had always been my recommendation that if you feel well enough to travel and your doctor says you can, then do it! Don't put it off as tomorrow may be too late, I know as I've been down that path on too many occasions.

Chapter Five.

Time's running out, but I'm able to travel.

Friday 6th April 2001

Appointment today at Worthing Hospital's day ward for Pamidronate. Had lunch there on the ward and was out at 1 P.M.

I accepted an invitation from my European Convention Bureau friend David to attend a reception on board an iron-plated sailing barques moored in St Katherine's Dock in the heart of London's Docklands. They served exceptionally good canapés, plenty of wine and good company made the day very memorable particularly as it was on a unique sailing vessel.

Following our nautical adventure, we ventured further into Docklands and made our way to the recently opened ExCel conference facility. It's huge, we were well received and had fun travelling on the DLR (Docklands Light Railway) although I think it may prove a little irksome when they hold the International Boat Show in January 2004 instead of its present venue at Earls Court which is so convenient to get to and the DLR is barely able to cope with anything other than low density passenger movements.

As I'm quite well at present, we take advantage of that fact and embark upon another holiday, the date 20th April 2001 and set off at 11:00 from the railway station at Shoreham by Sea and arrive at Gatwick at 12:00 noon. We checked in and made our way to the private lounge to enjoy their hospitality until 13:45 at which point someone shattered our peace and announced that our flight was about to board. We took off at 15:00 and arrived at Naples airport who still use the old Aeronautical Club di Napoli building as its arrival hall. It's a bit archaic, but the efficiency can't be questioned. In next to no time we had our luggage and were escorted to a transfer coach for our short journey to our hotel, the Hotel Dauphine at Marciano, seven kilometres outside Sorrento.

We arrived too late to eat in the dining room and were served a buffet meal in our room whilst we unpacked. The hotel had been built into the side of a hill overlooking the romantic isle of Capri. There was a small cove and even smaller 'beach'. From the water the hotel was almost undetectable as it blended in so well with its surroundings, a triumph in Town and Country planning, if indeed any exists in Italy, which I often doubt. The entrance foyer on the ground floor was guarded by a decidedly less than fierce Alsatian called Cretzia (Creature), who at a drop of her petticoats would roll over expecting, no, demanding that her tummy was tickled. The bedrooms were beneath the entrance foyer on different levels each with access to a terrace or garden. Our suite had two balconies with magnificent views across to Capri, the island that Gracie Fields made her own and having seen it in all its glory, I can fully understand why, it's simply beautiful.

On the Sunday morning following our arrival, we caught the local train, The Circumvesuviana to Naples, it runs around the bay and offers good views of Mt. Vesuvius and Pompeii and is excellent value at around £3 return. We were advised to be diligent whilst on the train as it's where the locals congregate and pick the pockets of tourists who are unaware of the potential hazards, fortunately we encountered no such problems. However as street crime is rife in

Naples, extra care was always needed, one of guests at the hotel told me that they were subjected to an attack, his wife was wearing a thick gold choke chain which caught the eye of a young thief who used bolt croppers to cut it from her neck, she bore the marks of the cutter to prove it, she should have taken the advice of the tourist police and kept her jewellery concealed. The local 'hoods' can spot the difference between a real and a fake Rolex watch at a hundred paces and would call out 'Hey Professori, fake Rolex', not wishing to have his social status being held in doubt, the wearer would often reply, 'No it's not, it's real' and have it stolen anyway! After a pleasant dinner, we adjourned to the cocktail bar but alas, they didn't have any olives, can you imagine that, we're here in a country where olive trees abound, the hotel is surrounded by olive groves and the hotel doesn't have any. The very next day we caught the transfer shuttle bus into Sorrento town and headed for a delicatessen to buy a large jar of olives for the barman, he was almost as appreciative as our fellow guests. From Sorrento's Harbour Piccolo, we caught the fast catamaran ferry service to Capri and thought the island was wonderful. A slight swell on the water made some of the passengers a little queasy, but to hardened sailors it was all part of the trip. There is much to see in this part of southern Italy and no visit can be considered complete until the Amalfi coast has been explored. We used local transport to visit Positano, a hopelessly pretty village hanging onto the edge of the cliffs. The bus ride was interesting as most people wanting to see the spectacular views would sit on the right hand side of the bus which caused it to lean violently around the twisting bends with nothing but fresh air between the bus and a sudden drop into the ocean. Those standing in the aisles, two deep were treated to an even closer view of the sheer drop. Positano is definitely somewhere I would revisit, but I'm not quite so sure that Naples would hold my attention for a second visit, unless it was by cruise liner pulling into the art deco liner terminal. The city has some really delightful buildings, but for me it's too cosmopolitan, too awash with crime to feel comfortable and far too noisy. A travelogue of Sorrento follows and a personal account of a distinguished local Anglophile who just loves to meet people in his marquetry shop and to sell them something if at all possible too.

'See Naples and Die'. (Under the wheels of a Lambretta!)

The Greeks first settled in Sorrento followed by the Romans who called the town Surrentum, or the 'City of Sirens', not police or fire engine sirens, which seem to wail constantly, but voluptuous apparitions who steered vessels on to the jagged rocks for which this coastline is notorious. The town, perched high on a cliff above the harbour, faces Naples and Mount Vesuvius across the Bay of Naples.

There are two designated beach areas, both situated by marinas, the main bathing activities take place from the purpose-built bathing platform at Marina Grande. The other harbour, Marina Piccolo, is used almost entirely as a passenger ferry terminal with boats plying to and forth to; Capri, Naples and Ischia, a smaller but no less popular island than Capri. The Roman emperor, Augustus swapped Ischia in 29BC with the Greeks for Capri, he obviously could appreciate its grandeur. Many tribes and nations have subsequently laid claim to the island, now it's the marauding tourists who rule triumphant. There is no promenade at Sorrento, sea vistas are from the elevated squares or hotel terraces fifty metres above the harbour. But the best view in town which can be had for the price of a cup of tea, is from the 'Circolo dei Forestieri' or Foreigner's Club which is situated behind the Tourist Information Bureau. Run by Michelle, an English lady, who married an Italian, Armando Alviani, the establishment offers tea and lunches during the day and dinner with jazz concerts in the evening. Fifty years ago, the club was the exclusive domain of the gentry, but happily now is open to all in need of refreshment, and occupies a privileged position with magnificent views across the bay.

The town is busy and vibrant, but still retains an old world charm around its cobbled streets which lead off from the main square, Piazza Tasso. The streets are narrow and flanked by tall buildings, the ground floors of which are shops, small marquetry workshops or cafés. Amidst all the hustle and bustle of this popular area, the visitor can still find a quite oasis like the cloisters within the Chiostro di San Franceso, just a few yards from another viewing terrace with an extensive panoramic view across the bay.

Conveniently, the bus and railway stations are close together just off the main thoroughfare, Corso Italia. But rather inconveniently bus travellers are unable to pay their fare on board the bus and have to buy tickets from tobacconists and then self-validate the ticket on board the bus. The railway station is a terminus and the Circumvesuviana train runs frequently to Naples, with stops along the route. The journey takes about an hour. En route, the train passes the stop for Pompeii, close enough for the ruins to be seen, although it also serves the modernised city beyond the famous ruins. English pensioners are able to gain free admittance to the ruins on presentation of their passport, not even Hampton Court Palace offers that gesture. Some visitors may prefer the less commercial and more intact city of Herculaneum, as Pompeii is very much a reconstruction according to how the builders imagined it and not the archaeologists. There is an abundant use of RSJ's and descriptions of the former use of the buildings which are pure fantasy. The streets are huge stone slabs, rutted from the cart tracks and any visitor can't fail to be impressed by the sheer awe of the ruins, even though much of it resembles a Lego kit with buildings re-created from the left over stones found during excavations.

There are few places where you can walk through streets built 500 years before the birth of Christianity. Pompeii was devastated by an earthquake in AD62 and restoration had hardly been completed before the city was destroyed again in AD79 when Mount Vesuvius erupted covering the whole area in volcanic ash from which it never recovered. Excavations were commenced by Charles of Bourbon, the King of Naples, in 1748. During his reign, he rallied against the English who had colonised the island of Capri in 1808 and witnessed their surrender in the Villa Rossi near the small port of Marina della Lobra, 5km south of Sorrento.

Much has been written, or even sung about the beauty of Capri, it is all true. It is a truly remarkable island, which is made even more magical by the fact there is only one way of getting there and that's by boat. It is a journey of about half an hour, if taken on the fast catamaran service. For a more genteel crossing, the steamer takes fifty minutes and is less likely to induce an attack of mal de mare! All the boats leave Sorrento from the Marina Piccolo, from 06:30 am and the last boat back is 21:00. However, if it doesn't run for any reason, the only way back is to take the ferry to Naples and get a taxi home at a cost of about £100, so always build in a time shock absorber when planning to visit Capri! From the ferry boat terminal in Marina Grande, Capri, there are several methods of reaching the town perched high above the harbour. You can take a bus, ride on the funicular railway, ride in style in a cabriolet taxi, or do what the locals do and walk. Half way up the steep steps that cut into the very heart of the town, is a small shop run by a small Italian woman who is raking it in from the sale of bottled water and other aids to recovery as if they are going out of fashion.

Transport on the island is fairly unique as it is apparent that it never seems to rain as all the cars are open-topped, even the buses resemble the charabancs of the 1930's and are open-sided, except for the bus service that runs from Capri town to the higher town of Anacapri. Here the bus company employ 'pushers' just like the Japanese railway system to ensure the maximum amount of people get on the bus which then laboriously plods its way up the steep and winding road to the higher town where there is a chair lift to the upper slopes of the mountainous rock formation. Although it may not rain in Capri, the top of the mountain is often shrouded in mist blocking out the wonderful views. Capri town is full of designer clothes shops in which the seriously rich can indulge themselves and despite the fact that the town receives many daily visitors, it is comparatively litter free. Electric buggies transport essential supplies to hotels and carry guests' suitcases along the narrow lanes between the buildings, reminiscent of the baggage carts at an airport.

In the church of San Michele, founded in 1719, there is an impressive tiled ceramic mosaic which covers the entire floor, not unnaturally visitors are not allowed to walk on it. There are a series of planks running around the periphery ending at the ornate alter. It's worth the climb to the first floor viewing gallery to be able to see this fine masterpiece in its full glory. The walls are covered with paintings from famous Neapolitan masters, the church should be on every Capri visitor's list. A much hyped and publicised area is the Amalfi Coast, the views from the elevated coast road are dramatic and considered to be some of the most scenic in Europe. Travellers with a nervous disposition should avoid sitting on the right hand side of the vehicle, particularly if it is one of the buses which regularly ply between Sorrento and Amalfi. So popular is the route that people take the bus just for the ride, rather than visiting a specific town like Positano where buses are not allowed into the town centre and stop on the roadside many hundred feet above the town. A small shuttle bus is allowed however and is well worth the few lire fare to avoid the lung bursting trek back up to the bus stop. Don't forget to buy your ticket in the tobacconist's shop in the town as you can't ride the bus unless you have one and this route attracts the attention of ticket inspectors who will impose an immediate fine of approximately £60 if you're caught without. Positano has a pleasant beach with a bathing station and a small quay from which a fast catamaran runs to Naples. The town is paradise for painters, who depict the brightly coloured houses hewn into the hillside with consummate skill. Although expensive, their paintings are a permanent reminder of a visit to this delightful town. There are just as many restaurants as there are painters and the town boasts several 5-star hotels with absolutely magnificent coastal views and a tariff rate to match.

Naples, just across the bay from Positano and Sorrento, is the major city and capital of the Campania region of southern Italy. Like any large commercial centre, Naples is a mesmerising confusion of roads and shopping streets with arcades through which Lambrettas ply in any direction they think fit. Riders of any age from 12 to 92 weave their way through the hordes of visitors and residents alike, it is not unusual to see a family of four including the family dog traversing the back streets that make up the city's residential area that most visitors should avoid during the hours of darkness. Areas of note within the city are, the Art Deco liner terminal which still has many cruise liners calling into the port en route to other Mediterranean destinations and the old fortress with its cloistered quadrangle. A fresco depicts the fort used as a barracks and training yard, made securer against the outside world by a pair of huge fortified gates.

Slightly away from the fort towards the city centre is the Teatro San Carlo with its impressive palladium style columns, gilded foyer and auditorium. Across the road from the theatre is the world renown Galleria Umberto, a vast under-cover arcade with four transepts emanating from a central piazza with cast iron and coloured glass atrium. Erected in 1905, the gallery is seen as a forerunner of today's shopping malls. There are offices on the first and second floors and impressive colonnaded entrances to the shops on the ground floor. The airport at Naples is operated by British Airports Authority (BAA) who have collaborated with the tour operators to ensure that outgoing passengers' luggage is pre-checked and transported directly from their hotel and placed on the aircraft. This saves the necessity of checking in with suitcases and the next time you see your luggage is on the carousel at your destination airport, well done Naples!

Whilst in Sorrento, we met Franco de Nicola, whose personal profile follows.

Franco de Nicola.
Four Generations of Marquetry.

Standing in a side street opposite to St Paul's church in the centre of Sorrento, sits a double-fronted shop with the appearance of gentle obsolescence. It has probably looked like this for the last fifty years and no one cares because it is accepted that Francisco's, or Franco's shop looks like that, and will always look like that, in his life time anyway. Franco's trade is not apparent from the fleeting glimpse that passers by give. They see old chairs with partly completed oil paintings resting on them, a dresser unit with newspapers dating back to the last millennium, carefully laid out as if to protect the surface of the wood which hasn't seen polish, yet alone wood stain in Franco's lifetime. From deep inside this unlit shop, emerges this sprightly octogenarian, a self confessed Anglophile who inherited the business from his father Carlo de Nicola, the grandson of the business founder who first applied his marquetry skills in the nineteenth century. The business, the furniture and the dust has been handed down from generation to generation and would be lucky to survive another change of ownership within the family.

Fluent in English, taught to him at school in his native Sorrento, Franco seizes every opportunity of greeting English visitors in his shop and is proud to have his photograph taken with them, which he adds to his considerable collection together with post cards from all over England from his newly made friends. There is no evidence of any marquetry pictures being made on the ground floor of his 'showroom', the workshops are upstairs he adds. But there is silence. He probably does just enough work himself in the evening when the showroom is closed. There is a small display of jewellery boxes and pictures, inviting potential new friends in for a chat. If he sells something, you are his friend for life, if you just admire his work, he treats you like a long lost friend.

Franco will readily explain the intricate fabrication technique involved in producing one of his masterpieces which comprise four layers of different wood veneers, glued together with his favourite bonding agent, fish glue. The wood is bought from local sources, his favourite and most widely used woods are; burr walnut, olive, ebony, briar, rose, orange, lemon and cherry. This selection of wood gives him all the colours he needs to produce his goods. He will undertake commissions for monogrammed items, these he knows have an appeal and receives his money upfront so he is manufacturing for a purpose, rather than 'just in case'.

There are numerous shops selling marquetry in Sorrento, many have their work shops on display, but none of them have the same appeal as Franco's genteel showroom. Should you ever find yourself in Sorrento with half an hour to spare, visit him at 35 Via Tasso just off the main shopping street. You will be assured of a warm welcome and the chance to purchase a small item, say a musical box, from his limited range. Also don't forget to send him a copy of the photograph of him with you. He takes off his English cloth cap to reveal a full head of dark brown hair and has an endearing smile which is not quite so full or as brown as his hair.

Tuesday 1st May 2001

I'm not sure, but I think I may have slipped out of remission and that my cancer's returned! Had a bit of a temperature and saw Dr Roques in his clinic at Worthing Hospital where bloods were taken for analysis and antibiotics given to stem the infection. Temperature rose to 38.2° by the evening.

Friday 4th May 2001

Appointment in day ward for Pamidronate. I have a cough and my chest and ribcage hurt through coughing. If I'm well enough, we wish to have a short break with our friends in Dorset, I hope I'll be alright but you can never tell with this condition.

Tuesday 8th May 2001

I do feel all right and well enough to travel. Dr Roques gave his blessing to our trip so off we went to Swanage. I continued to cough much to the annoyance of others I'm sure. Ribs still hurting greatly which may well be because the cancer has returned.

With our friends, we headed off to Dorset and stopped for crab sandwiches by the quayside at Wareham. The sun was shining and everything in my world seemed all right. Our stay in Swanage was at the three star Best Western Grand Hotel situated high on the headland overlooking the bay. The scenery in this part of Dorset is both spectacular and undulating, so many travellers just pass straight through Dorset on their way to Cornwall and never really stop to enjoy its beauty.

Monday 28th May 2001

No news from the hospital regarding my blood test, so it's assumed that there's no immediate problem. Dr Roques gave his consent for me to fly to Geneva to accompany my friend on his stand at a travel trade show, just to get me out of the house and doing something interesting.

David and self caught the Easyjet flight from Gatwick at 12:45 and despite several bad reports that the airline had been suffering from recently concerning delays, surly staff and indifferent attitude by the cabin crew, we found the whole experience very straight forward and the personnel could not have been more pleasant. As both my friend and I like to sit by a window, it pays to be quick off the mark once boarding has been announced to get the seats you want as they are unallocated. My friend would invariably tap me on the shoulder and point out something he has seen which might have interested me, in reply I would invariably state in more than just a whisper, 'I don't know who you are, but if you don't stop pestering me I'll report you to a flight attendant!' He enjoyed the banter and it kept the other passengers amused too. As is often the case, Geneva is wonderfully warm in May and the weather on this trip was no exception. I was feeling a little tired from 'people watching' all day at the Palexpo, situated in the lee of the airport which quite uniquely straddles both France and Switzerland. I returned to our hotel for a short nap before being taken to dinner as guests of the Italian Tourist Board on board the paddle steamer *Helvetia* moored on a pontoon on the shore of Lac Leman (Lake Geneva). Whilst there I met the Israeli Tourism director who invited me to a sumptious breakfast banquet the following morning at the Crowne Plaza hotel near the airport. It was the best breakfast feast I had ever sampled and saw a short promotional film expounding the virtues of visiting that country. Sadly with all the troubles both past and present it was an up hill struggle for them, but I enjoyed their hospitality. So much so in fact that I attended the following day and took my friend with me, who being a vegetarian was in his element with the hundred and one meat free dishes on offer, we were late for the trade show. We ate very little throughout the day and enjoyed a cheese fondue and rösti at the Petit Chalet in Geneva's city centre in the evening, it was our last night there and marked it in style.

I was still tired, but had survived the trip quite well and glad I went along for the ride for I don't know if I'll be well enough in the future to do it. Having packed my bag, we arrived at the airport at 12:45 for another straight forward flight home. I was on the train to Shoreham by Sea by 16:00, nothing could have been easier.

Monday 4th June 2001

More bone-strengthening infusions at Worthing Hospital's day ward. It really has improved my tolerance to pain and is helping me enormously, thank goodness. On the following Thursday, I was off with my sailing buddy, Alan for another sailing weekend at Poole. We had a great sail even though it was quite blustery. We took a rest at the Sandbanks Ferry café with coffee and sticky buns before sailing the five miles back to Rockley Point to prepare ourselves for the evening's entertainment routine of snooker and takeaways, predictable or what?

Friday 15th June 2001

Experiencing an awful lot of back pain today, my ribcage is mighty uncomfortable too. It's either muscle pain from the rigorous sailing yesterday, or the myeloma has returned!

Saturday 16th June 2001

Goodness, I'm in so much pain today I can hardly do a thing without wincing! I dosed myself up with Southern Comfort laced coffee and got out onto the water after lunch with a reduced sail area to make life a little easier for me, I didn't stay out long and had to come in because the pain was too much to bear.

Sunday 17th June 2001

We managed a last sail in the morning before showering and packing ourselves and the boat up to return home by 17:00. I had an invite to our daughter's for dinner as long as I didn't turn up covered in seaweed. Trips away have been a constant talking point since my illness and I was given every encouragement by our daughter to continue doing so. I mentioned that my sister had made her apartment in Florida available to us whenever we wanted, so it was decided that at Christmas we would do it. We had only ever travelled in Europe, so America would be a totally new experience for Julie and myself.

Tuesday 26th June 2001

In quite a lot of pain today especially around the shoulders but I don't have a temperature so there may not be a problem lurking.

Saturday 30th June 2001

We are off on holiday again! Why not, the doctor says that there is no reason not to go and a rest from all my other activities might ease the pains I've been experiencing in my back, ribcage and shoulders. We travelled with our non-flying friends again, so it was the usual shuttle bus down to Dover Docks to board the ferry bound for Calais. To avoid queueing in the cafeteria, we take a leisurely dinner in the restaurant and enjoyed the peace and quite for a hour. The sea was a little choppy, so eating didn't really interest all of our party. We arrived at a Holiday Inn on the outskirts of Paris at 23:30 feeling very tired and retired to bed immediately. After an early breakfast we took the coach to the Gare du Lyon via a scenic route taking in the River Seine. Paris is beautiful at any time, especially at seven o'clock on a summer morning when the sun is rising and reflecting off the buildings.

We board the Trains Grande Vitesse (TGV), which on this occasion is a double decker train. It's so convenient and fast, we reach Toulon in just four hours. It's hot down there in summer and this is only the first week in July. There was a 45 minute coach transfer to our hotel, le Grande Hotel in Bormes-les-Mimosas, an unbelievably pretty medieval hill village just half an hour from the Cote d'Azure. The hotel had been in the same family since its construction over a hundred years ago, might even get round to redecorating it one day, but don't hold your breath! The two areas of natural history common to this immediate region of France are; Cicades (Cigales) who rub their back legs together each evening at dusk hoping to attract a mate. The other species is the Hoopoo bird, it's not an accusing question amongst other birds, but a tree dwelling bird related to the owl family. The Nightjar spends all night hoopooing in its attempt to attract a mate. The village shops can supply artefacts of any known material, colour and scent just as long as its Cicada-shaped. I didn't see one wax candle in the shape of a Hoopoo bird!

It's even hotter today, Monday 2nd July at 33°, we Brits aren't used to it, so we do what all Brits do when their hot and at the seaside, we roll our trousers up and paddle in the sea. The small town of la Lavendou has a small marina with various shops and restaurants and a ferry service to the nudist colony at Siestre Levant. The same boat serves two of the other islands in the bay, we stopped off at Port-Cros and met an interesting British man from our home town in Sussex. A travelogue covering the area and a personal profile on John Wilsher follows.

PROVENCE, I'VE BEEN AWAY TOULON!
A travelogue by Peter Berry.

It must be nearly forty years since I last visited southern France, not surprisingly, things have changed a little! The greatest change that has occurred, is the speed at which the holiday maker can be on the Côte d'Azur. Forty years ago it took me four days to drive down there. Admittedly, it was in what was affectionately called "a sit up and beg" 1953 Ford Popular and the route took in all the well know watering holes such as Paris, Dijon, Lyon, Grenoble, Digne les-Bains and finally through Grasse to Cannes. Ever tried to find a campsite in Cannes? Quite an epic journey for those times and flying was not a considered option as it was too dear and besides, what do we do with all that camping gear?

Flying was not an option on this trip either as our group of six, had decided to "let le train take le strain" and board the TGV (Train à Grande Vitesse) from Paris to Toulon. Because of the recent improvements to the track, the journey time has been shaved from five, to four hours. It is the train's twentieth birthday this year, the very first train stands on a plinth outside Strasbourg.

There has been much written in the travel pages recently of the efficiency and other qualities of this high speed train, so I will not preach to the already converted. I will just say that four hours is better than four days in my book and anybody else's. For much of the time spent thundering through France's Grand Massive, the traveller could be anywhere in England, particularly the verdant pasture lands of the West Country. Fields with grazing cattle look pretty much the same anywhere, except for the preponderance of Charollais cattle which are quite distinctive, being nearly pure white. The traveller is not afforded a casual look at the countryside, as most of it rushes past in a blur so things may tend to look the same.

It is only when the outskirts of Avignon come into view, that the passengers start to feel that they are approaching both civilisation and more importantly, a climate that is associated with the Mediterranean. On the newly built station, which was our T.G.V.'s only stop en route, the waiting passengers were wearing flimsy clothing and gave those of us on board the air conditioned train our first impression of just how hot it was outside! On arrival at Toulon station, a transfer coach was ready to whisk us away to our chosen destination of Bormes-les-Mimosas approximately forty-five minutes drive. More time would have been appreciated in Toulon which is France's second largest port and is home to much of the Navy. The city was important in Roman times for the production of purple dye. Conche shells were boiled to produce the colourant used in the manufacture of Papal garments.

So many improvements have been made to the waterfront, which now has wide terraces and the usual array of cafés with their chairs and tables almost constantly occupied and water taxis offering the customary harbour tours. Hitler invaded in 1942 and the French scuppered their fleet of seventy-five warships, which, after the war, took ten years to clear.

The road up to Bormes from the main highway, is steep, winding and very busy and because of the medieval town's enormous appeal, it attracts visitors and local alike. Ninety-nine percent of the visitors drive there, with the odd one percent made up of those hardy racing cyclists, who are in training and use the hill as their testing ground. We, on the other hand could regard ourselves as "residents", albeit just for a week, but nevertheless we were staying just a few yards up the hill at the Grand Hotel, a building of faded grandeur and furnished "in the French rustic style". The current owner, Mme Marie-Laure Gouttepiffre, is the grand-daughter of the founder, who had the hotel built in 1903. It was a grand hotel in those times, with sweeping lawns cascading down from flower-bedecked terraces with the gentry parading in their finery, or so the oil painting in the secondary dining room would have us believe. The terrace is still there but used partly as a car park and the lawns have long since been built on for dwelling-house development, probably to provide working capital to keep the hotel running. As it is, le Grand closes down for the winter from November until April. Despite its rustic charm (this means no air conditioning or modern plumbing), the hotel is ideally placed for exploring Bormes' numerous alleys and covered walkways. Probably the most photogenic street is, Rue Rompi Cuou (literal translation is 'Bum Breaker' because of its steepness and slippery stone steps). Bougainvillaea and oleander shrubs adorn every inch of walls that the traders have not covered with samples of their merchandise.

Views from the hotel to the sea, just six kilometres away, are truly magnificent. The Iles d'Hyeres just ten kilometres off the bay can be seen easily as can the small ferryboats that ply between them. It is only a thirty minute trip to Port-Cros, the smallest of the three and has no made up roads, only compacted gravel tracks on which the Mini-Moke from the island's only hotel, Le Manoir, plies the handful of privileged guests to and from the ferry. If it's total seclusion you seek, this hotel is your answer, if it's night life you're after, don't come at all. There is a fort on the hill, built in 1580 which we British blew up in 1793. This no doubt gave the French another reason for claiming not to get on with us. They have never forgiven us for setting fire to their saint, Joan of Arc.

The nearest large town to Bormes is le Lavandou which has a wide seafront and promenade, a marina from which the ferry across to the islands leaves and a treacherous footpath that hugs the coastline round to St Claire which boasts yet another sandy bay with a backdrop of pine tree clad hills. The marina has numerous eating places and what could be more relaxing than taking a two hour lunch over a bottle of rosé and bowl of moules?

A somewhat larger marina is found at St Tropez, named after a Roman legionnaire Torp who was banished from his fort for spreading Christianity. It is alleged that he was set adrift in a small boat with a dog and chicken for many days. As neither he nor the dog had eaten the chicken by the time the boat was washed up in a small bay, it was regarded as a miracle and the soldier was canonised. Thus the town takes his name, St Tropez. Once the visitor is away from the gin palaces moored as "tight as sardines in a tin" along the harbour-side, the town has a number of narrow streets, churches, shops and restaurants.

The price tag on the clothes in the shops will give some idea of the huge amount of wealth that the area attracts. Italian chic is very much in evidence here, presumably emanating from its origins within the Holy Roman Empire, as was Nice before it was overrun by the French.

A much newer town is the one created out of swamp land just south of the ancient town of Grimaud which was once owned by the Grimaldi family, who at that time lived in Genoa before moving to Monaco. There are the remains of an eleventh century castle there and the church of St Michael, that pre-dates it by three centuries. The new town, called Port Grimaud by its founder and architect François Spoerry, was commenced in 1966. It covers an area of 100 hectares and has 2,500 houses lining the seven kilometres of canals which are up to four metres deep. With safe mooring for 3,000 boats, Port Grimaud is always a popular place to visit, whether it be by road or sea. You can even moor your boat alongside the church of François d'Assise. There are spectacular views from the top of the church tower, which collects a five franc coin for the privilege.

No visit to Provence would be complete without seeing Aix en Provence, which is rumoured to have 365 fountains (one for each day of the year). Some are easier to find than others as they range from huge edifices of Victorian proportions occupying the whole of a traffic island, to small drinking fountain size. One is purported to be the Fountaine Chaud, or hot spring, which it isn't. However the minerals in the water are certainly different to all the others and have encouraged the growth of a thick moss-like plant all over it. To see fields of lavender swaying in the hot Mediterranean air that most people symbolise as being typically Provençale, a visit to Alpes-de-Haute-Provence, is required.

There is very little of it in the coastal plain region, except for in the shops where it abounds. Visitors can take home as souvenirs; pomanders, lavender honey, nose-gays and just about anything else that has ever been in contact with a lavender bush, including the area's favourite insect, the cicada or "La Cigale". This creature makes an unholy din as it rubs its back legs together like a cricket, however it is much larger, more like a stag beetle with huge lace wings. They are supposed to bring good fortune, they certainly do to the shop keepers who sell; stuffed ones, soap ones, candles, lapel badges and much, much more!

One thing which they don't stuff is the other noisy resident of Provence and keeps you awake at night, the Nightjar or Hoopoo bird. It has a metallic ping of a call, not unlike the sound your smoke detector makes when the battery is low. Many non-naturalists would be delighted to see stuffed versions of this in the shops too.

I will revisit Provence and not wait another forty years before doing so. The TGV was fine except you have to board it in Paris, which of course means getting there in the first place. I found a delightful, small airport at St Tropez Le Mole into which Crossair and Lufthansa fly and I reckon that has to be the easiest way of getting down there. Now, where's that tent?

End of travelogue.

A Life on the Ocean Waves
A personal profile of John Wilsher

How many people do you know who have at sometime or other uttered those well used words, "I'd like to just sell up and sail off into the sunset?" They want to abandon society and all its falsehoods and live the life of an itinerant sailor. I have met such a man, he did just that over forty-five years ago and would never go back to his previous life. He would find it too difficult to fit in and wouldn't be happy in any case.

John Wilsher has been living on his beloved boat *Pindoe* since 1956 and is currently moored in a small harbour in the south of France. In his totally nonchalant style that has become John, he announces that "I have no permanent home, I live wherever I moor up, my present postal address is, John, Port-Cros, France. " Unbelievably, mail reaches him at this address, it may take several weeks, but what's the hurry?

I met John, who is an affable, sun and wind tanned itinerant sailor whilst on holiday recently on the Côte d'Azur. I took a ferry boat from the Provençal town of Le Lavendue to the small island of Port-Cros, one of the Ile du Hyeres archipelago. Lunch time beckoned, so my wife and self adjourned to a harbour-side café for lunch, not expecting to share a beer or two with such an interesting character as John.

We dined on moules and thick rustic bread and were acknowledged by a very English, "Good afternoon", there was a slight French inflexion which comes from living for nearly fifty years amongst French citizens. We gave a polite return salutation which broke the ice for further conversation to take place. Establishing from what region of England we were from, it transpired that John had lived within a mile of where my wife was born in Hove on the south coast, the conversation became more intense. Born in Hove on the 16th December 1931, John lived for a number of years in Lorna Road where his grandparents ran a sub-post office and grocers shop. He moved from there with his parents when they bought a lock-up grocers shop in another part of Hove. "I lived in Buckingham Avenue, Shoreham by Sea" he announced, less than half a mile anyway from where we live. I researched his claim in the Shoreham library's copy of Kelly's Directory and found an entry for Walter Wilsher at number six, this was John's father.

John had trained as a boat builder and lived close to where the ship yard was on Shoreham Beach. He converted many of the former Motor Torpedo Boats, (MTB's) into house boats when it became fashionable to have a sea-side home. There was no shortage of buyers for the converted boats as Shoreham Beach boasted a film studio and attracted the film industry's big names immediately after the war. Some of the boats are still moored in the river on the north side of the shingle spit that has now become a housing development. Sadly many of the boats are now rotten and are breaking up only to be replaced by former Thames lighters which already show advanced stages of corrosion. John said that he made a lot of money stripping the brass fittings of the boats, including the propellers known as 'screws'.

When recounting his lifetime's association with boats, it was established that at one time, he had owned the Netley Abbey boat yard near Southampton and specialised in repairing traditionally built wooden boats. He sold up in 1956, took to the water in *Pindoe*, named "Beautiful" in Greek mythology, a 23 foot sloop of larch on oak construction. Built in 1932 at Portsmouth and weighing two and a half tons, she is a well founded vessel which has transported John around the Mediterranean for many a year.

I asked him for how long he had lived in this idyllic setting and how he came to be there in the first place. He replied, "I needed to effect some general maintenance whilst moored up in Cannes. I could do everything there, so set sail for the boat yard in England. My route was to round Gibralta and up the Bay of Biscay into the Atlantic Ocean and into the English Channel. I was under provisioned and called into Port-Cros for water and supplies and have been here ever since, that was 1994"

With a safe harbour and pretty much ideal weather conditions, John sees no real need to up anchor and continue his voyage. Without putting to sea and braving the notoriously rough Bay of Biscay, he doesn't need to effect the repairs either. July generally sees a brisk wind blowing about these parts and boat owners who have not 'battened down the hatches' securely, find themselves in need of John's skills as a boat builder to effect repairs. His wages come in the form of returned kindness, as most boats are owned by restaurateurs and the like, who will keep John supplied with beer and fresh food. He is a simple man with simple habits, when we first met I asked him if he lived here, his reply was, "I exist here!"

We were seated on chairs that he had made and at the table he constructed, the list of wooden fixtures was endless. Stephanie, a pretty, young French girl brought us fresh supplies of beer. "Many the times I've touched up her rubbing strakes" John informed me, "She's got beautifully rounded lines and sits well on the bottom". I couldn't have agreed more with him more. "She's about sixty years old" he informs me, I would have said more like eighteen and fresh out of college. I think we were talking about different things.

Time means nothing to John, "I get up when I want, eat when I'm hungry and drink when I'm thirsty." He has no watch, mobile phone, or satellite tracking system, why should he? He isn't going anywhere. He's got fresh fish for supper, a few beers 'in the till' and no responsibilities apart from looking after Stephanie's stern gear. I wonder if he needs an assistant?

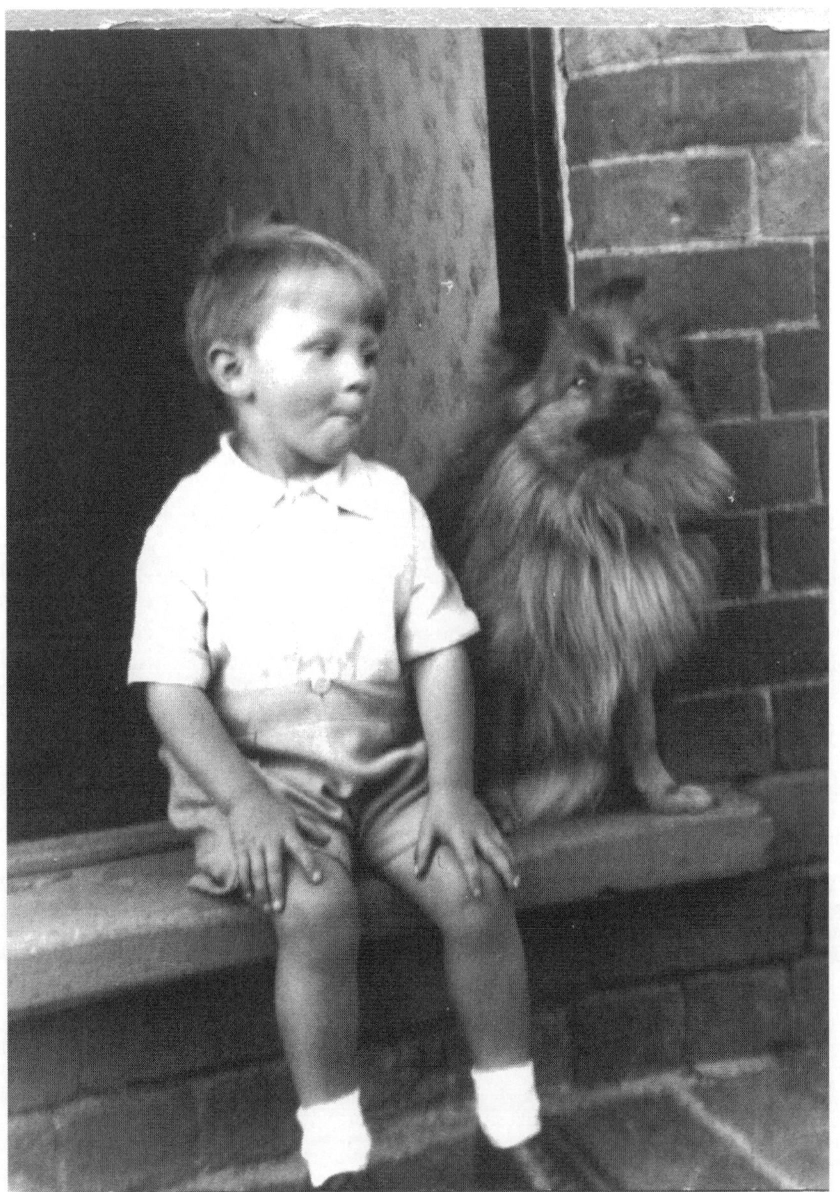

Peter at 30 months old with Tony. (on doorstep).

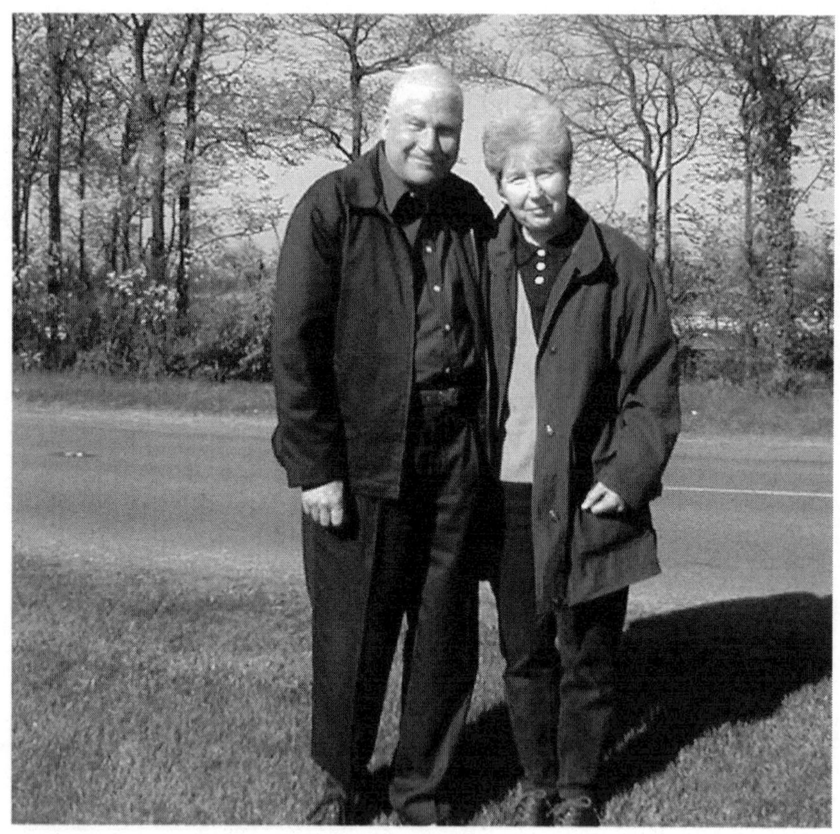

Peter and Angela.

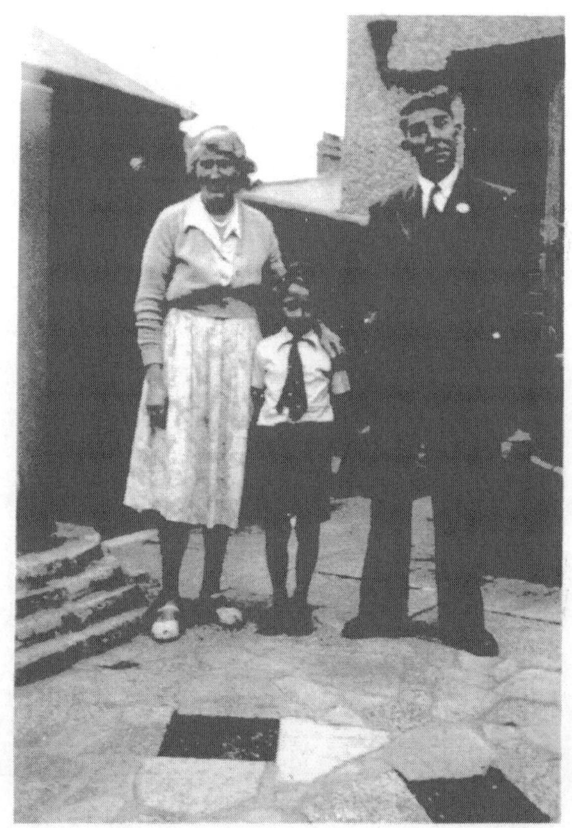

Peter and Parents in Portsmouth.

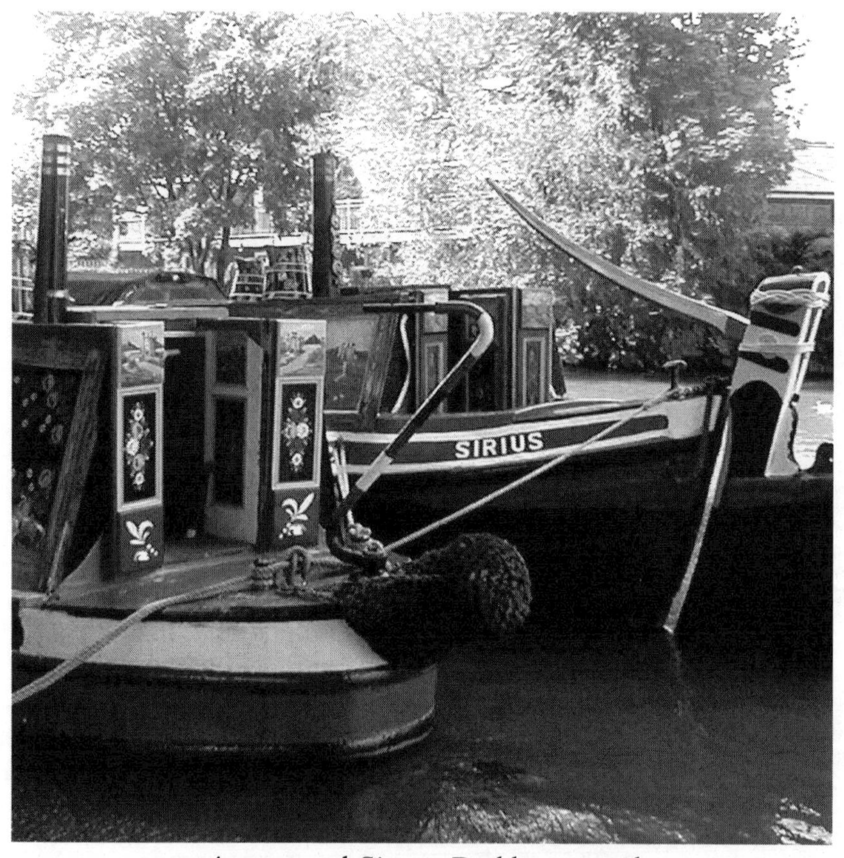

Arctueus and *Sirus* at Berkhampstead

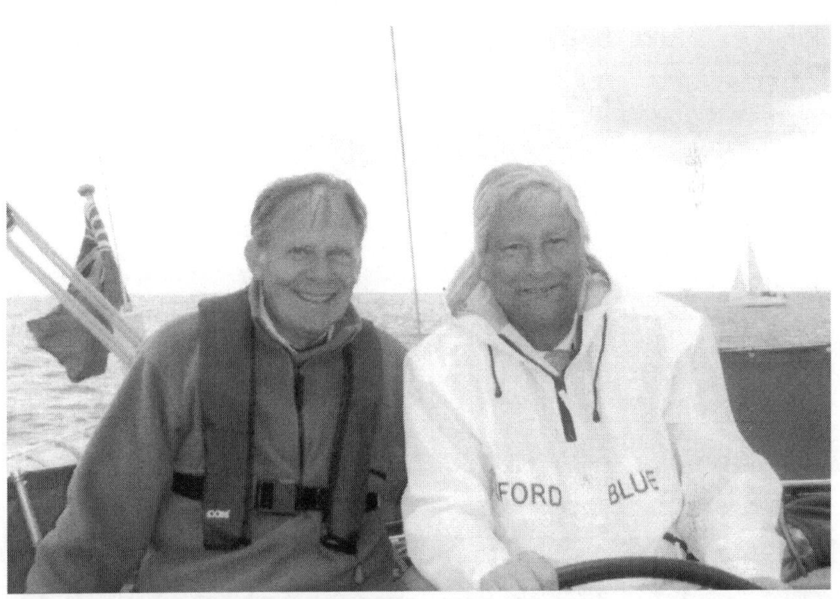

Alan & Peter aboard *Cascade.*

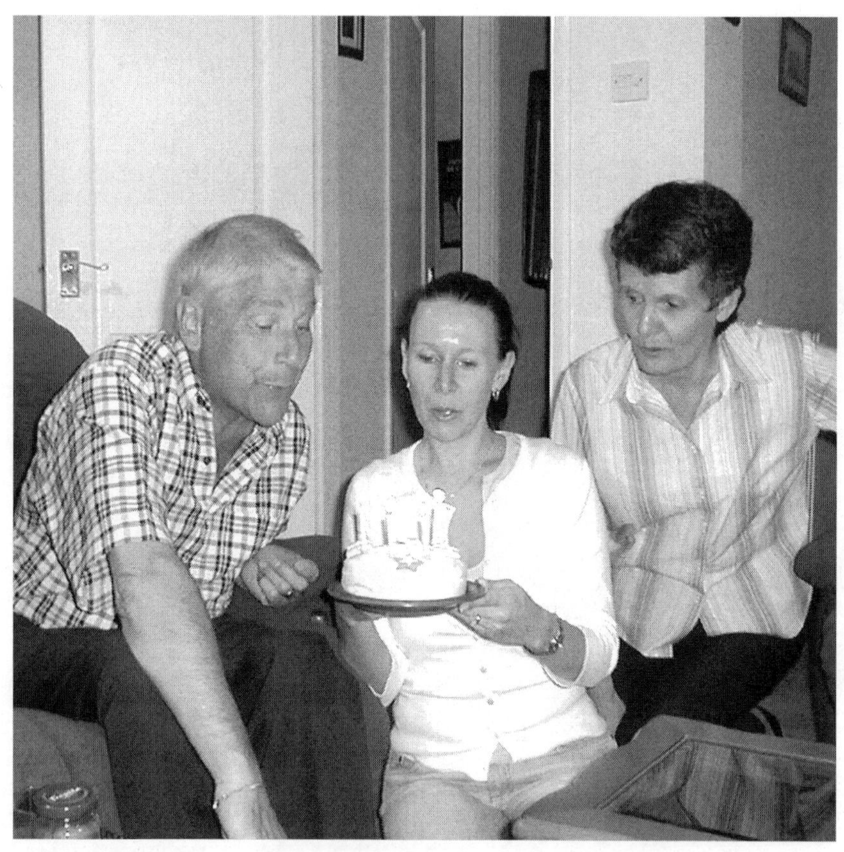

Peter's 60th Birthday at home.

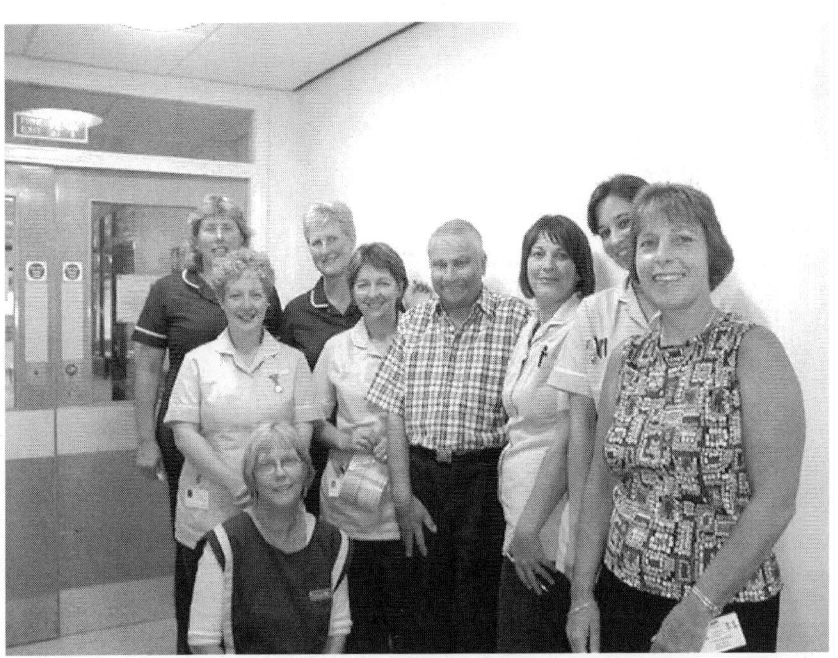

Peter's Birthday with his personal nurses.

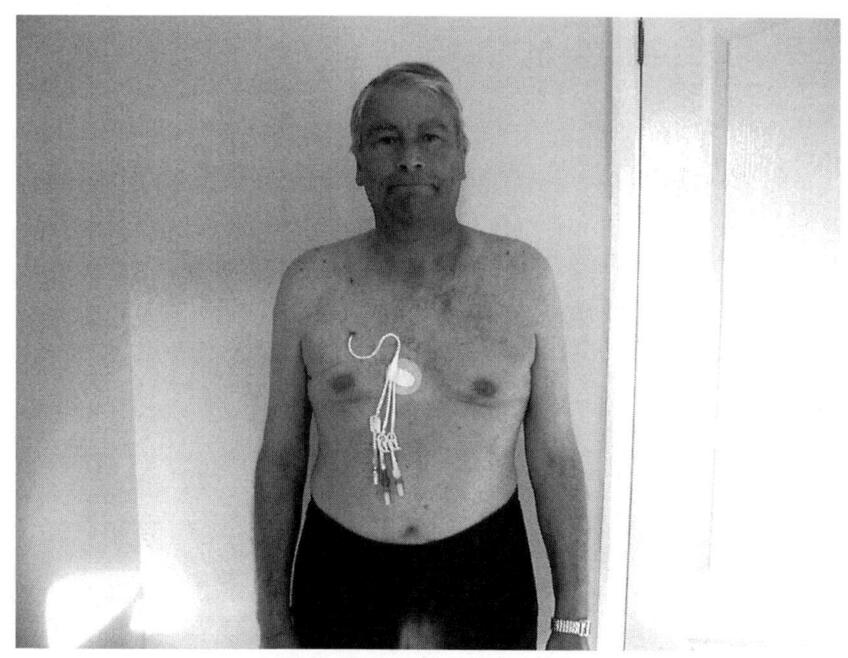

Peter with his Hickman Line.

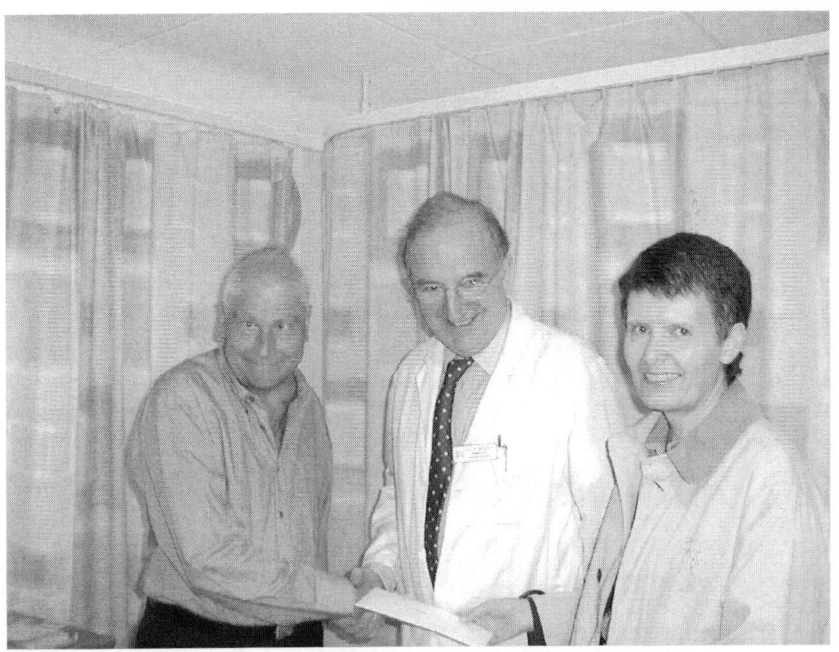

Dr. Roques 65th Birthday

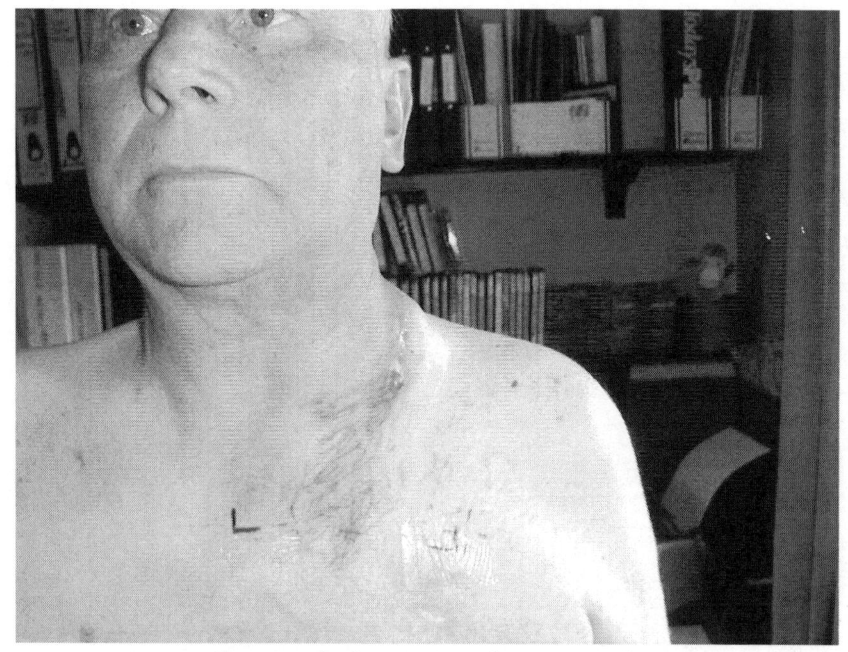

Peter marked out prior to being zapped.

Chapter Six.

The Winds of Change.

Monday 9th July 2001

I'm back from holiday and survived without the need of medical attention whilst I was away. I immediately attend a prearranged appointment in the day ward for more Pamidronate to strengthen my bones, the treatment lasts the usual 90 minutes, give or take half an hour whilst I'm waiting to be hooked up to the drip or chatting to my many friends in the ward, both patients and nurses!

The airline tickets for our flights to America have been bought and paid for, I felt that at long last we were on our way to Florida, in the good ol' U S of A. I was now hoping that I'd continue to feel well enough to make the trip. Our travel insurance company, American Express had reinstated my full cover to include my Multiple Myeloma and so I felt confident to venture outside of Europe where there is always the reciprocal health care agreement covered under the E111 form which has been used to good effect on a previous holiday in Italy.

On a more local basis, we travelled down to Portsmouth Harbour with our friends on the train to visit the Historic Dockyard which included a tour of the famous ships from bygone years. The place was seething with French students, about a hundred stood alongside Nelson's flagship, HMS Victory and sang La Marseilles at the top of their immature voices, I'm not sure if this was a protest because we defeated Napoleon's fleet, or an impromptu concert, but their indifference to the English was obvious.

Thursday 26th July 2001

A busy day medically today, it starts off with a visit to the day ward at Worthing Hospital for Pamidronate followed by an appointment with my specialist, Dr Roques in his clinic. He suggested that I undertake a series of x-rays to monitor my condition and check to see if there was anything obvious that was causing my continuing pains to the back and ribcage.

Saturday 28th July 2001

Although not a medical matter in the strict sense of the word, I nearly had a heart attack when exposed to the following series of events.

Whilst waiting in my car at traffic lights on the A27 at Lancing, West Sussex, a truck and six wheeled trailer came out of a side turning that lead to the municipal rubbish dump, it took the corner too fast in an attempt to beat the lights and toppled over alongside my car. The entire contents of the trailer spewed out and smothered my car in all sorts of debris including old bed mattresses, bushes, bikes and bedsteads! I was lucky to escape injury, just very shaken by the experience. The car however was extensively damaged and the road closed for several hours whilst the lorry was righted and all the rubbish put onto another lorry. I can't pass this spot now without thinking back to that day which could have ended in tragedy. It would have been a pity to see all of Dr Roques good work over the last three years destroyed in a millisecond. Although I am a member of the National Union of Journalists, I didn't have a camera or notebook with me, so I left it to the police to interview all those involved and take the photographs, a fine reporter I turned out to be! The press pass issued to me did however allow me access to some local aviation orientated shows. At Shoreham Airport there was a helicopter and vintage car show, Rotors and Motors where I met several interesting people. My writing course dictated that I interview as many people as possible to gain journalistic skills and it's surprising what people will tell you if you announce you're from the press, albeit freelance. I didn't sell any of my articles, I did it for therapy and to broaden my horizons and get me into places that otherwise would not be available to me. It was true to say that my life had been enriched by my membership to the N.U.J. I'd worked for 40 years without belonging to a trade union and now that technically I wasn't working I was a paid up member of a union! I had never attended any of their meetings, using the Press Card purely for my own benefit in getting into events that I would previously not have been allowed access to. I found that the credibility of holding a Press Card was a boost to my confidence and I should always be grateful to their management for allowing the union to grant me membership. One such event was Eastbourne's 'Airbourne' flying display held each year in the Summer around July time. Although this event is open to the public without charge, I was entitled to sit in the press tent and interview the pilots and the Red Falcons parachute display team. I was also invited to a flight in a Bell Jetranger helicopter which took me along the coastline to Beachy Head and its lighthouse. Whilst at Airbourne, run in conjunction with the Civil Service Motoring Association (CSMA), I met Pierre Picton who owns the original Chitty Chitty Bang Bang, a nineteen twenties 'boat back' Bentley valued at half a million pounds and a Laurel and Hardy lookalike pair who call themselves Haurel and Lardy who have a genuine model T Ford imported from America and used in one of the Laurel and Hardy films. These people were delightful to talk to and their presence added a great deal to the day.

Monday 20th August 2001

I'm in absolute agony today. The pain in my side is excruciating, I can't sleep at night and wonder what on earth is going on, although I have a pretty shrewd idea, I just hope I'm not correct in my assumption.

Friday 24th August 2001

I'm having to take extra pain killers to combat the pain it's so severe, I feel very drugged all the time and quite tired through sleep deprivation caused by the pain.

Tuesday 28th August 2001

My glands are up and my throat feels 'peppery' a sure sign of impending trouble like an infection or at least a common cold. I ring the specialist who prescribes a course of antibiotics. I told him that the pain in my ribcage is severe, he will monitor the situation over the next few days and give me advice as to what will happen next.

By the following weekend, the prescribed drugs had done their job, I felt much better and the pain was easing. There was another air show to attend as a freelance journalist, this time at the annual Royal Air Force Association (RAFA) show at Shoreham Airport. I was able to sit in at the pre-flight briefing sporting my press pass and met members of a display team who invited me to ride 'buck shot' in the vehicle which tows a flat bed trailer on which a Piper Cub aeroplane lands whilst we're hurtling down the runway at seventy miles an hour. I took some great photographs and interviewed the team, none of this would have possible without my membership of N.U.J. and representing the freelance press.

On the Sunday following the show and still feeling well enough to get out and about, we travelled with friends for a short break on the Isle of Wight which is quite close to us. Catching the Wightlink ferry from Portsmouth across to Fishbourne, we arrived in Shanklin's old village for our four night stay. It gave us the opportunity of exploring picturesque towns and villages such as Godshill, Bonchurch, Bonniface Down and Ventnor. I took my new 'toy' with me, an Olympus digital camera, the decision to buy was almost forced upon me as I'd spent about seventy pounds buying disposable cameras and having them developed and printed for the two air shows I'd previously attended. If I was going to pursue journalism as an interest, I had to find a more economic method of taking the photographs, the only answer was a digital camera. I took a series of pictures of the hotel's staff and gardens and offered to show the proprietor my efforts on his new wide screen television which had been delivered earlier that week and cost him eighteen hundred pounds. He was quite impressed until we were unable to restore the set to its proper function. He informed us that his mates were due round in half an hour to watch football and if the TV wasn't working by then, we'd all be in deep water. Thankfully a few prods and pokes of the right wires in the right holes restored his set and our credibility, we didn't show any more pictures on his set after that.

Friday 7th September 2001

I'm due to attend a routine check up at Hammersmith Hospital's haematology Dept today. I tell them I've been experiencing severe pain in my ribcage. They take the customary blood samples but they didn't reveal anything, I'm very surprised that they didn't because usually pain means there's a problem somewhere.

After attending the appointment, we continued 'up country' to Watford which for most southerners is the demarcation point between north and south. As I was born in the Midlands, Watford is still quite a long way south for me. We stayed at the Best Western White House Hotel in the town centre and very pleasant it was too. We were both surprised at how large and pleasant Cassiobury Park was and how near it is to the town centre. The following day we met the owners of my grandparents' former boats, Arcturus *and* Sirius *over a nice lunch beside the Grand Union canal at Whitwell before driving back via Heathrow to book a hotel for the eve of our trip to Florida in December.*

Monday 10th September 2001

The pain in my ribcage is still quite severe and I'm rather concerned about it now, it seems to have been with me for some time and just will not ease up. Having more tests to see if it reveals anything, this will confirm or deny any suspicion about what is happening to me. It's also my 57th birthday, the best present I could possibly have is to feel well again.

Tuesday 11th September 2001

A bleak day for the whole world as terrorists fly airplanes into the World Trade Center in New York. The world will never be the same after today.

Thursday 13th September 2001

Received a letter from Worthing Hospital advising me that I am to attend an appointment for an MRI scan. It transpires that the senior radiologist at Worthing, being aware of the pain I was suffering, re-examined my x-rays and wanted to compare the state of my back and ribcage against the MRI scan that was conducted in 2000.

Pain or no pain, it didn't stop me getting myself out and about if I possibly could. Using my press pass, we attend a helicopter trade show, Helitech at Duxford Aerodrome in Cambridgeshire before travelling across to Norfolk to meet up with my sister whose birthday it is today, the 24th. We stay at a delightful and rather superior bed and breakfast establishment, a Georgian manor house at Watton Green just outside Norwich.

Thursday 18th October 2001

Further bad news, Dr Roques believes that my Multiple Myeloma has returned, I'm no longer in remission, I've relapsed! This comes as no great surprise as I've been in quite some pain for the last six months. Although I could never ignore it, I have tried to 'soldier on' and not just stay at home and contemplate my navel. This relapse co-insides with the 30 month prediction given Dr (now Professor) Jane Apperley at the Imperial College London following my first period in remission. Our disappoint is obvious after so much has been done to put me into remission in the first place.

Saturday 20th October 2001

I have to attend a flu jab clinic at the local GP's surgery. I am one of those considered to be 'at risk'. Both my wife and daughter have one also as they could pass on a virus to me if they picked anything up. My immune system is suppressed and I need to avoid further problems.

Monday 22nd October 2001

Have got to conduct a urine save over the next 24 hours so that the specialist can check for any increased levels of para-protein. This is an indicator of by how much the myeloma has returned.

Tuesday 23rd October 2001

Attending an appointment with the specialist who will conduct a bone marrow biopsy which is yet another test to establish the presence of the cancer cells in my marrow, it's the 'acid test'. I'm sedated as I don't want to feel the auger gouging into my hip to extract the viscous fluid, I have a number of biopsies and always opt for sedation. Whilst there, I'm to have a Polio and Typhoid inoculation too. I will not know the outcome of the biopsy for about a week, so perhaps one last chance to travel if I feel well enough. The specialist says, I can go if I wish.

The tour operator, Voyages Jules Verne sent through one of their last minute 'flyers' suggesting we can travel to Morocco to take advantage of cancellations following the atrocities of 9/11. It appears that several passengers were rather sceptical about travelling to a Moslem country in the wake of the terrorist attack. We knew the risks and also that it may have been the last chance to travel for quite some time, so we went before I have to notify the travel insurance company that I've definitely relapsed. Tony Bennett should have sung, 'I left my pain in Marrakech' rather than heart in San Fransisco for as soon as I stepped onto the tarmac in Morocco, the pain in my back and ribcage just disappeared as if by some form of magic. Being free from pain was such a relief, I could sit beside the hotel's swimming pool and even at ten o'clock at night the air temperature was 88° and made me feel good. The air conditioned bedrooms gave us some respite against the heat which was obviously doing me a power of good. After our 'welcome meeting' we were put onto a coach and driven to the old part of town, the Mhedina and taken through the souks. Words couldn't describe how we felt and reacted, it was as if the clock had been wound back 2,000 years and we were walking along narrow passages in which Jesus Christ would not have looked out of place.

We looked on in awe at the grubby eight-year-old boys hammering bits of metal into a roughly hewn shape that would eventually be an artefact for sale in some other traders shop. They in turn look on in awe at one of the members of our party, who made all her own clothes and dressed in the style of a nineteen thirties film star. The locals had never seen anything like it before and were convinced that she was either still a film star or a princess. Neither side could believe the incredulity of the sight they were seeing as 'Binky' was neither a princess or film star, just an eccentric who never moved a yard without her make up case, even wannabe princesses have wrinkle lines.

Having seen the Giralda Tower in Seville, we were now looking at the original on which it was based in Marrakech, the Koutoubia. Close by is the bustling Jamaâ El Fna (square of the dead) which was noisy, dirty chaotic and wonderful. There were snake charmers, jugglers, acrobats, organ grinders with monkeys and any number of stalls selling local food stuffs and hot meals all at ridiculously low prices. I would have loved to have sampled some of them, but daren't for fear of picking up a bug of some sorts. I restricted my food intake to that served by the hotel, at least I knew that there's a reasonable chance that it's alright. To get away from the relentless hustle and bustle of the city, we hired a personal chauffeur and old Mercedes 'Grande Taxi' for the day with two other guests and head for the Atlantic coastal town of Essaouria. The road to the coast is straight for 100km, goes round a rock and then straight again for the last 70km. En route we saw goats up trees eating the argon nuts, the oil which is extracted from the kernel is an essential part of the process in perfume manufacture, and a camel train. The town had been spruced up for the imminent visit by the country's king, Mohammed VI. If it didn't move, paint it white. After a thoroughly enjoyable week and meeting wonderful people, we flew home on Wednesday 31st October, I made sure I didn't collect my pain on the way out. A fuller travelogue on Morocco follows.

MOROCCO
The Ancient Kingdom of Mogador

How can anyone prepare you for your first contact with this ancient country and its wonderful people? They can't, you just have to see it for yourself and revel in its glory. The land is one of extreme contrasts and assaults your senses in every way possible.

Although just off the Straits of Gibralta and extending eastwards along the Mediterranean coastline and down the west side of the Atlantic coast, Morocco is in Africa and its culture is immediately self evident. It is reflected in the costumes and appearance of its inhabitants, seventy-five percent of which are Muslim. Their daily call to prayer is paramount to their very existence, however, Morocco is a tolerant country and respects other religions.

In the vibrant city of Marrakech, there are churches devoted to all denominations, schools are segregated, but sit side by side in perfect spiritual harmony. If ever there was a race of people who deserved the title of the most industrious nation, my nomination would not extend to the northern European countries which we immediately consider to be worthy of the title, I would choose the Moroccans. They are very good at manipulating inert pieces of metal, into any object that is needed. In the totally overwhelming souks that are found in central Marrakech, there are eight-year-old boys hammering out and stamping pieces of metal, the finished article may never be seen by them, but their contribution to the process is energetic and totally committed.

Every Peugeot 205 that was ever made and subsequently died, has been transported to Morocco. It has been rebuilt by the side of a dusty road without the assistance of any sophisticated equipment, and made to run again. It is subsequently sprayed in a Sahara sand colour, given a number painted on the side and used as a Petite Taxi. In Marrakech, there are 1,500 of these little marvels dashing about all over the city and the prices charged are no more than a Pound for just about anywhere in the city. Larger Mercedes taxis, or Grande Taxis are less numerous, unmetered and still so cheap as to make travelling without one churlish. A hired Mercedes and personal driver for an eight hour day for four people travelling a 350km round journey was the equivalent of £40. The driver thought he was conveying royalty, we thought we had a personal chauffeur.

The Moroccans are very proud of their Royal ancestry, currently, King Mohammed VI reigns and is highly revered, particularly by the Marrakech residents, as the King often chooses to reside in his palace there, rather than in the official palace in the country's capital of Rabat which has a population of 1,500,000. Marrakech was the capital, any many still regard it as such, although there is little chance that its title will be restored. Founded in 1602 and part of an empire stretching from Toledo, Spain, to Senegal in West Africa, Marrakech is known as The Pink City as it takes on the colour of the local earth used in much of its construction. Other imperial cities, once the country's capitals were; Fes and Meknes before losing their crowns to Rabat. Fes is the most ancient of the imperial cities and was constructed in the 8th century. It is purported to have more history and mystery than any other city in Morocco. The other former imperial city of Meknes, echoes the splendid and grandiose building projects that were commissioned by the country's then ruler, the Alauite Sultan Moulay Ismaol who ruled from 1672-1727. He was in awe of Louis XIV's palace at Versailles and wanted to emulate the extravagant style of architecture. One of the most fascinating parts of daily life in Marrakech, is activity around The Djemmaa-el-fna square. There are snake charmers, dancers, storytellers and fortune tellers. Many locals eat there from the dozens of small kitchens set up at dusk. Two of the most popular ancient palaces to visit are; the El Bahia Palace with its numerous courtyards and gardens, and the 16th century Saadian Tombs which house the remains of the rulers of the Saadian dynasty. The higher the ridge on top of the tomb, the greater was the importance of the occupant. The most revered of all the rulers, was Ahmed el Mansour who ruled between 1578-1603. He built the Badii Palace with its wonderful gold, onyx and marble features, all traded for their own weight in sugar. Morocco has many elements which make up its fascinating and varied features, it has; the Sahara Desert, the Rif and Atlas mountains and covers a total of 275,000 square miles, which makes it larger than Texas! It produces dates and bananas, as well as tomatoes and green stuffs including mint from which the local brew of Moroccan Whisky is made, it's just mint flavoured tea, no alcohol. The climate is diverse enough to encapture all elements of agriculture. It is also unique in the fact that the Argana trees, which produce a highly sought after fruit containing a kernel rich in Argon oil and used in the manufacture of cosmetics, is only found on the outskirts of Essaouria, just off the Atlantic coast. The fruit can't be harvested by traditional "cherry pickers", mechanical devices on tractors because of the thorny nature of the tree. The locals do however train their goats to acquire a taste for the fruit and when the stone is passed through the animal, it is collected and sold for oil extraction. They don't put that fact on the label!

Morocco was formerly divided between the French and Spanish colonies, but became independent in 1956, except for a contentious enclave in Melilla in the north of the country which is still in Spanish control. The Spanish influence in the architecture is high and the Koutoubia Mosque Minaret in Marrakech, has an identical one in Seville, known as the Giralda Tower which also dominates the sky scape of that city. Morocco's first head of state in 1956 was Sultan Mohammad V, who changed his monika to that of King until his death in 1961 when his son Hassan II succeeded. On his death, the new King is Mohammad VI who retains total power over the country and appoints the Prime Minister.

Thursday 1st November 2001

Attended the previously arranged appointment at Worthing Hospital for another dose of Pamidronate and to see Dr Roques who, as expected confirmed our worst fears that the biopsy had revealed that the Myeloma had definitely returned. I was therefore booked in and admitted to hospital on Sunday to enable the treatment to commence.

Sunday 4th November 2001

Checked into hospital at 15:00 hrs in preparation of a new Hickman line being inserted the following day. I have to have a special antibacterial bath to cleanse my skin of all exterior bacteria.

Monday 5th November 2001

Another special bath just to make sure no trace of bacteria remains and I've to be ready for my operation at 08:00 hrs. I'm not allowed to eat anything, just have a cup of tea to keep my fluid intake up. There's a delay and I won't go to the theatre until 14:00. I was wheeled back onto the ward by 16:30, not too bruised and battered, just a bit sore around the entry point.

Tuesday 6th November 2001

Chemotherapy due to start today, Vinchristine and Doxamoxin (VAD) delivered into my blood stream via the Hickman line through a pump contained in a 'bum bag'. This time there is a new supplier of the chemo who have put the liquid in a tube that is twice as large as the previous method and quite conspicuous in use. Having a litre bag of saline fluid to hydrate me to avoid further kidney damage.

Wednesday 7th November 2001

I'm now over-hydrated and need a blood transfusion to restore matters. I'll be allowed home today but will have to return to hospital tomorrow.

Thursday 8th November 2001

Attended the day ward for two units of blood, group 0+, it'll take until 17:00 to go through which means I get to eat one of the hospital's delightful lunches. They conducted blood tests and gave me the results as follows; White cell count 7.2 against a normal of 7-8, Haemoglobin of 8.4 against a normal of 14, Platelets of 174 against 199 and Neutrofils of 5.9 against 5-6. So all in all, I'm nearly up to scratch.

I contacted American Express Insurances Services to advise them that I had relapsed, subsequently they withdrew my fully comprehensive, worldwide cover for matters connected to the Multiple Myeloma. The upshot of this, was without full cover in place, I couldn't afford the risk of flying to America at Christmas, so all our plans had to be altered dramatically.

Saturday 10th November 2001

Hickman line needs flushing, attended day ward, tomorrow they'll take out the securing stitches.

Tuesday 13th November 2001

The day starts all right, but by lunchtime I'm shivering so the hospital is advised who want me to pack a bag and report in immediately. Given antibiotics as a precaution and sent for x-rays to check my lungs in case of Pneumonia.

Wednesday 14th November 2001

I'm tachicardic (rapid pulse) with a temperature of 38.2° and a sore throat.

Saturday 17th November 2001

Things appear to have stabilised and I'm allowed home after lunch with various antibiotics. Starting to experience some hair loss from the VAD chemotherapy.

Friday 23rd November 2001

A busy day health matter wise. Seeing local GP here at home at 10:00 for him to get up to speed with my condition. District nurse coming at 11:30 in order that she can flush my Hickman line, however it transpires that she is not qualified to do so and we have to go into the day ward. Day ward nurses train my wife, Julie to flush the line herself and change the end pieces (bionectors), she did very well. If we do flush the line at home there is less risk of picking up an infection from the hospital.

Monday 3rd December 2001

Second VAD chemo due today, have to attend day ward for the pump to be connected and whilst there to have another infusion of Pamidronate.

Wednesday 5th December 2001

Face and body now quite bloated by the steroids, chemo making me feel very sick. Knowing that I was likely to feel even worse within the next few days and not really wanting to do anything other than just sit quietly, 'quiet lifing' as I called it, I visit an old friend, Patrick at the shop he worked in near Worthing's town centre, he approached me as if I were I stranger and doesn't recognise me at all because I've bloated so much I look a Weeble. Even when I talked with him, I don't think he really realised it was me despite the fact that we have been close friends for over 40 years, are godparents to our respective children and he and I worked in nearby stores in Guildford. He at Pimm's who had a furniture shop and marine branch where Flick worked and was one of 'the gang' who used to attend summer barbecues on the meadows close to the river, and me at Kinch and Lack, the 'Gentleman's Outfitters'.

Wednesday 19th December 2001

Julie rings me on my mobile phone, the hospital want me to go in immediately! She'd already packed a bag for me and collected me from a reception I was attending marking the 'Passing Out Parade' of one of my friend's helicopter training courses. When the day dawned, I had no idea this is how it would end up. I was at a hotel just outside Shoreham airport perimeter to attend a buffet lunch for a young lady who was to be presented with her helicopter 'wings'. She and her sponsor Dennis flew the Hughes 300C into the hotel's car park. It was quite an emotional moment, I would loved to have stayed, but when the hospital says 'jump' you have to jump.

Thursday 20th December 2001

I've got an infection in my Hickman line and it has to be sorted out quickly or risk having to have the line removed. I'm given three lots of the antibiotic Vancamicin through the line to flush any infection out of it. May go home tomorrow if all's well.

It was not quite 'Three Men in a Boat', it was more like 'Three boating men in a Bed', I'll explain. The ward into which I was placed saw me in the middle bed, on my left was Tony who has the same medical condition as myself and was a power boating enthusiast (his wife, Flick, I knew in Guildford 40 years previously) and on my right was an estate agent friend and sailing buddy, Chris Ennis who I'd known for 20 years. The chances of the three of being in adjacent beds must have been very long odds indeed.

Saturday 22nd December 2001

Problems developing during the day, having to be re-admitted at 16:00 hrs for more Vancamicin, hoping not to be in hospital over Christmas. I may get away with going in every day rather than be an in-patient.

Christmas Eve 2001

As promised, attending Erringham Ward at Worthing Hospital at 09:30 for more Vancomicin, should be out by noon.

Christmas Day 2001

In hospital again by 09:00 for more antibiotics, what a way to spend your Christmas! I expect to have my Christmas lunch in hospital, no crackers, no party hats and definitely no alcohol. It's not going to be the happiest of Christmases for any of my family, especially as we should all be in Florida together, still, there's always next year. Hope to be 'sprung' by tea-time.

Thursday 27th December 2001

Having to attend hospital, yet again and been on the day ward by 09:00 hrs for blood tests then on to see the specialist. Feeling much better in myself now that the antibiotics have finished, the cure can sometimes be worse than the cause.

Monday New Year's Eve 2001

It's New Year's Eve and I'm having to attend hospital again, it seems never ending. I've got to have another course of Chemotherapy VAD through my Hickman line. On top of that I've got to have another infusion of the bone-strengthening agent, Pamidronate and don't expect to be out before tea-time. I'll see what the canteen at the hospital can rustle up for me.

What a way to have spent New Year's Eve after last year's celebrations in Funchal, Madeira. There were some fireworks let off by the local pub, but no where near as impressive as those in Madeira where the town's Mayor spends a substantial amount of his annual budget on the pyrotechnics. What we saw locally was more like the five shilling selection box I was bought as a boy from Boswell and Carver's in Rugby.

Tuesday New Year's Day 2002

Another year of treatment ahead of me, feeling reasonable except for the effects of the chemotherapy. Starting another course of steroids so I expect to bloat up again and to feel ravenously hungry, except I don't really fancy much in the way of food. It has to be bland with no onion, everything tastes metallic from the chemo, it's not very pleasant.

Saturday 5th January 2002

Time for the VAD pouch to be disconnected and the line flushed, I'm feeling quite poorly today and know it'll get better once the VAD has gone through my system, in the meantime, I feel very bilious and I'm fighting to keep food and fluids down.

Wednesday 9th January 2002

Yet another course of steroids due today, I've bloated so much I feel as if my head is going to explode, my sight is distorted by the shape of my face being altered through bloating and I can't do my trousers up, having to wear jogging bottoms. Although I feel a little better today, I've developed a cough which, if left unchecked could turn into Pneumonia again. The hospital suggest I come in for some Ciprofloxacin, yet another antibiotic to counter the effects, but I don't have a temperature which is a good sign.

Sunday 13 January 2002

Feeling very poorly through having antibiotics but it's the weekend and not much support is available at the hospital today. I'm coughing but it's not productive and there's no temperature, I'll risk waiting until Monday before I report to the day ward.

Monday 14th January 2002

I decide to contact the hospital who say pack a bag and come in for check ups, don't know yet if I'll have to stay in, I might get away with being dosed up and sent home later in the day.

Tuesday 15th January 2002

Some hopes of not being admitted, I was checked in and advised that I've got a chest infection and must have yet more antibiotics intravenously through my Hickman line. I'm shaky, my chest rattles, I'm tachicardic and neutropenic, as if this wasn't enough, I've got to have a bone marrow biopsy, yet another hole drilled into my hip to get to the marrow. Having to use a nebuliser to help my breathing, don't know when I'll be well enough to go home.

Thursday 17th January 2002

Chest infection under control, breathing's better, temperature normal and cough still not productive, so all being well I should get out of hospital by tea-time today.

Thursday 31st January 2002

I wish I could say that I felt ok, but I don't. I'm still shaky and feeling very weak. I report into Dr Roques who recommends that I be re-admitted to hospital to get me well enough for the imminent admission to Hammersmith Hospital for my second stem cell transplant using the reserve cells from the initial harvest. Whilst I'm in hospital I'm possibly to be given Pamidronate and a forth session of chemotherapy as we don't yet have a date for Hammersmith. A line swab is to be taken in case my rising temperature is being caused by an infection.

Friday 1st February 2002

I've got Chicken Pox! The last time I had that was when I was ten years old and passed them onto my sister who has never let me forget the fact. As I'm deemed to be highly infectious, I'm moved into a cubicle away from all other patients and notices are placed at the door stating don't enter unless under supervision. There appears to be some dispute whether I've got Chicken Pox or Shingles so the 'Pox Doctor' is to be called for to decide the matter. The nurses, most of whom are mothers know it's Chicken Pox without a specialist being sent for to decide whether it's Chicken Pox. Or not!

Monday 4th February 2002

I'm too poorly to have the forth VAD chemo, my Shingles/Chicken Pox is all over my head, trunk, chest and back, it itches like crazy and my temperature's up to 39.1°, it's a good job I'm in hospital. I'm going to have some Piritron through my line to ease the pain, I should sleep well as it's an opiate drug, the dissoluble co-codamol did nothing for me so the stronger drugs have been brought out of the medicine cupboard. I think my Hickman line is infected, the doctors are doing all they can to save it in readiness for Hammersmith.

Friday 22nd February 2002

Having been discharged from Worthing Hospital, I'm sent up to Hammersmith to see the specialist prior to being admitted, they know of all the problems I'm having and they want to see if I'm well enough to be admitted and made even more poorly! I saw a consultant who was definitely 'not up to speed' on my case, he didn't even know that I'd relapsed, didn't give us a lot of confidence and told Professor Jane Apperley of our displeasure. Still no definite date for admission to Hammersmith.

Wednesday 6th March 2002

Need to see the dentist to sort out any potential mouth problems before I have the high dose Melphalan chemotherapy. She refuses to scale and polish my teeth for fear of breaking the skin and letting infection in.

Monday 25th March 2002

No date yet for Hammersmith, now another problem has arisen, my Hickman Line is blocked. We can't get blood out of it and can't put any antibiotics or Pamidronate through it. Whatever the problem is, I've got to be re-admitted to Worthing Hospital as soon as possible. If the line can't be saved, at least I'm in hospital where they can remove it, but they'll try all the tricks in the book to save it for me. I'll have to be canulated to administer all the drugs as I've still got a temperature.

Thursday 28th March 2002

My line's unblocked, my temperature's down, I can go home!

Thursday 4th April 2002

Due to have another MRI scan today in Worthing, not too bad here compared with Hammersmith's old-fashioned apparatus. Feeling quite good now, but still no date for Hammersmith, it's getting frustrating as it's difficult to make any plans.

With nothing else to do, we decided that before I was due to incarcerated for a month in a 12 foot by 12 foot magnolia painted room in Hammersmith

Hospital, we ought to have another few days away somewhere. We decided to revisit my birth place, Rugby in Warwickshire and see my girlfriend Angela who I was going to marry when we were both eight years old. She and her husband Bernard made us very welcome and spent a nice day in their company. By coincidence, Bernard used to live in Braunston, the village that my grandparents lived in and operated Arcturus *and* Sirius *from. We revisited the docks and other old haunts including the school my mother attended, the village had grown, but was still recognisable.*

Whilst in Rugby, I showed my wife the railway line which is now a cycle path and the two bridges that I used to race the LNER's Master Cutler between. The following day we booked into Wharf Cottage, a nice bed and breakfast cottage by the side of the canal at Stoke Bruerne, opposite to the Waterways Museum. The owner's husband, David Blagrove used to work as a boy with my grandfather, Ike Merchant in the dock at Braunston. He remembers well the visit by the then, Prince of Wales who surprised my grandfather by swearing like a trooper after hitting his head whilst trying to get inside the captain's cabin of Arcturus*. Ike was purported to say that he didn't know that royalty knew swear words like that! Whilst at Stoke Bruerne, we contacted one of my other friends from the road in which I lived, Tony Clewett and his wife Julie who joined us for dinner in the adjacent pub restaurant where we recounted old times. He, Angela and myself were just some of the ten or so kids in the road that 'played' together some fifty years previously, he hadn't altered at all.*

Sunday 14th April 2002

The long awaited day has arrived, today I am to be admitted to Hammersmith Hospital for the second Stem Cell Transplant. Having to ring at 09:00 to ensure a room is available to me. A great disappointment, room not yet vacated by previous patient, must try again tomorrow.

Monday 15th April 2002

Still no beds, must try again tomorrow.

It has been very obvious that attempting to secure a bed up at Hammersmith Hospital is very difficult indeed. I phoned as instructed to ascertain the availability of a room into which I could be admitted, only to be advised that it had been allocated to a patient who was already an in-patient of the hospital. This required action being taken to ensure that a room would be available to both Julie and myself. We booked ourselves into another ward in order to be on hand when the bed clerk said there was a bed available in the cancer clinic, it seemed to work.

Tuesday 16th April 2002

Success! Although I haven't been allocated a room on a cancer ward, the bed manager says it's better to be in the hospital rather than 70 miles away, as in-patients will always take precedence over out-patients. We pack our bags and await collection by the hospital car service.

Wednesday 17th April 2002

We are told that I've been allocated a room on Weston ward in the relatively modern cancer centre, this is good news as it means we can get on with the treatment. Taking I/V steroids (Dexamethazone) which will mean more bloating and hunger pangs.

Thursday 18th April 2002

Today is our 32nd wedding anniversary, what a way to spend it! No cocktails, other than of drugs, pills and potions, no special dinners, only luke warm hospital food. But you get used to missing out on important occasions with this illness. It is also BMT (Bone Marrow Transplant) day minus four.

Friday 19th April 2002

The day is already in full swing at 06:30, I am receiving Cortizone and sickness cover for the chemotherapy treatment known as Melphalan, which I will receive later today. The dose will only be 140 mg compared to 200mg last time which made me very ill indeed. The reduced dose is either because I'm now four years older and not able to cope so well, or the Myeloma was caught in time and a lower dose is all that is necessary to knock it on the head. No one can really tell me the definitive answer. I've started to feel very tired. Had a visit from the dietician to advise me on eating a 'clean diet' whilst in hospital for the next four weeks and when I get home initially. No pepper, no shellfish, blue cheese or active yoghurt etc.

Saturday 20th April 2002

Still on a saline drip to hydrate me against kidney damage as the creatinine levels in my urine are still high. I can't afford to endure more kidney damage. It is BMT minus two to receive my stem cells back and I'm starting to feel the effects of the chemotherapy a little more today, it's making me feel very off.

Sunday 21st April 2002

BMT minus one today, I'm being monitored very closely to ensure that I'll be well enough to receive the cells back tomorrow.

Monday 22nd April 2002

BMT zero day, I get my stem cells back today, my temperature is checked and it's normal and although my throat is closing a little through mucusitis, it is no where near as bad as it was four years ago when my throat closed completely and I had to be fed intravenously. I'm to have another Cortizone injection against rejection of the stem cells, but as they are my own cells, there should not be a problem. Mine is an Autograft, rather than using donor cells known as an Allograft. The cells are due to be given back to me at 13:00 and apparently smell of oysters or sweetcorn, although I've never smelt them previously, but others can.

Wednesday 24th April 2002

It's my eighth day in hospital and due to have Vigam Immuglobulins to boost my immunity system which has been wiped out by the chemotherapy, I'm neutropenic. The pain my throat is tolerable and as yet there is no need to be connected to a diamorphine pump. Being on one's ok, it's the coming off it again that makes me twitch. I believe the expression is 'cold turkey'. As I haven't got any immunity at all, I pick up infections from every source. I've got a urinary tract infection and a skin flora which is a fungal infection, to be given all the necessary drugs of Telcoplanin for the cystitis and Clotrimazole for the flora.

Sunday 28th April 2002

The doctors ask again if I want to be connected to a morphine pump, they seem quite disappointed when I tell them I can cope without it. Feeling bilious for most of the time now, a mixture of the chemotherapy and the other drugs for my infections. Given Domperidome to quell it.

Friday 3rd May 2002

There's something else to be concerned about now, my Hickman line entry point is particularly sore today, there's some puss and it hurts like crazy when the nurse squeezes it. The infection will have to be identified and dealt with, I can't afford the risk of losing the line so close to completing my treatment. I'm also running out of available places on my chest for a new line to be inserted, so we must save it at all costs.

Tuesday 7th May 2002

A big step forward today, I'm no longer neutropenic, my blood counts have come up well, I've got some immunity back. I've been in hospital for three weeks now and will probably be here for another week. Temperature is up a bit at 38.2° so given paracetamol to bring it down which makes me sweat profusely and makes me dehydrated so will have to go on a saline drip to rehydrate me as a protection against kidney damage. I'm to be given two units of blood tomorrow to perk me up a little in preparation to being discharged next week. Hickman line is saved thank goodness.

Tuesday 14th May 2002

Exactly four weeks after being admitted to Hammersmith, I am to be discharged later today, after lunch probably once my stock of drugs has been made up from the pharmacy dept. We say our good byes to staff and patients and totter unsteadily to the transport dept. where the hospital car is waiting. On discharge my blood counts were;

White cells 7.2 as opposed to 5.9 on admission which is an indicator of how well I've responded to treatment. Neutrofils 4.3 as opposed to 5.6 so still some way to go there before back to normal, platelets almost up to par at 202, they were 199 on admission four weeks ago.

I could not get over how green and large everything appeared, I'd only seen four walls for a month and they were painted Magnolia, so anything with any colour in it was a real treat. The trees were in full leaf, people were wearing short sleeved shirts and not hospital green 'pyjamas' it was so good to be going home to the peace and quite of one's own home. It wasn't the treatment or the boredom that got to me, it was the hospital food, it was awful. The endless struggle to get warm, not even hot food from the temporary hostesses when the regular one was having a day off or on holiday was very wearing. I would complain that the meal was cold, only to be told that it wasn't when it left the kitchen twenty minutes ago, need I say more? The system was very nearly cracked after a while, we mentioned to the dietician that food was a problem and she recommended meal vouchers which could be exchanged in the cafeteria. However, as they cater for a largely Asian community, most of the meals were either curries, spicy this or that, or open salads which I wasn't allowed to eat for fear of picking up a food related bug as it wasn't considered to be on the dieticians 'clean diet' sheet. Eventually we abandoned the idea and my wife would walk into East Acton or Shepherds Bush to buy microwaveable meals from the supermarkets, that way I got hot meals that weren't spiced up.

Whilst I was recuperating, it was a question of 'quiet lifing' when I didn't feel I could do anything other than just sit in a chair and let the world carry on its business without my intervention. When I did start to feel more 'with it', I would take the opportunity of going for short walks to regain some muscle strength in my legs which wasted away to matchsticks. The park opposite the house gave me the opportunity of walking and sitting on one of the numerous seats when the necessity arose. I wasn't allowed in shops, on buses, in pubs, not that I had any desire to drink alcohol at all, the nearest I came to that was mouthwash which made me light headed anyway. There were regular visits to the haematology clinic at Worthing for check ups, the sheer fact that there are more germs to be picked up in hospital than just about anywhere else you can think of, didn't bear thinking about, but I got away with it, just.

Thursday 6th June 2002

I've to attend an appointment at Hammersmith as they have a vested interest in me. I am told by the specialist up there that all's well, the treatment has been a success and there's no need for me to go up again, let hope he's right! That news rather put a degree of finality to the proceedings, I had rather got used to a second opinion every other month or so since my first stem cell transplant back in 1998. I did ask whether it was possible to do yet another stem cell harvest to give us some reserve stock of stem cells, but it wasn't possible, two transplants are all they can do, I'd used up my allocated supply and that was it, no more. New procedures were developing all the time, so it was possible that other methods might have been available in the future if I needed them, we wait and see. My intention then was to put into practice what I had been preaching and take every opportunity of travelling. There was so much catching up to do since I was deemed to be in remission, which included travelling as often as possible and to visit all those relatives that should have had a visit but through circumstances, I hadn't had the opportunity. My diary was filling up fast. I estimated that I had approximately two years before I would relapse again, as remission doesn't last as long on subsequent occasions, so every single opportunity to get out and about was taken, for tomorrow it may not have been possible. That was always my dictate and I was sticking to it, I couldn't afford not to.

Chapter Seven.

New horizons.

American Express Travel Insurance would not re-instate full cover until I'd been in remission for six months, so a secretary at Hammersmith was primed to send them a letter stating that I was placed in remission on the 19th April and in 24 weeks thereafter, I was able to travel again. That brought me up to the 6th October 2002, with the first trip due on the 14th to Chicago. I was denied the chance to go last year, nothing was going to stop me this year, terrorists or no terrorists. That was my very first trip to America and I loved every minute of it. David and I stayed in New York at The Pennsylvania Hotel opposite Penn Station for one night which gave me the opportunity of doing the things on the tourist trail such as riding the subway downtown to Battery Park and catching the Staten Island ferry, going to the top of the Empire State building and seeing what is probably one of the most beautiful buildings in the whole of America, the Chrysler Building. I flew out from Newark Liberty airport the next day to Chicago, a city I felt immediately at home with, it had boats, an extensive waterfront and an interesting overhead railway system mounted on wooden piers with planking above street level, the whole thing shook when two trains passed at speed on the same section of track.

Following my return from Chicago, there was a brochure on the doormat from Voyages Jules Verne, inside was an offer to experience a river cruise down the Nile, we had often considered such a trip but were yet to do something positive about it, this then seemed an ideal opportunity to put right what we knew we should have done ages ago but never quite got round to it. It was ascertained that space still existed on the trip for November 2002, which we subsequently booked without further delay.

The Nile and all the towns and villages adjacent to it were seething with frenetic activity, it is more than just a main arterial thoroughfare, it's a way of life for many thousands of people. They bathe in it, drink it, do their washing in it, irrigate their crops and water their live stock, as a result there is a degree of prosperity along the river banks which is not as obvious elsewhere. The people, as with other Muslim countries, are wonderfully friendly and would go out of their way to be of assistance to you, they need the tourist's money and are expert in making you feel more than happy to give it to them.

A travelogue on the Nile cruise follows.

Tourism within Egypt is still suffering to some extent from the massacre on the 17th November 1997 when 58 tourists were gunned down by extremists at the ancient temple at Karnak on the west bank of the Nile near Luxor. That tragic event triggered a scepticism to travel to Arab or Muslim countries which was further fuelled by the atrocity of 9/11 in New York in 2001 when Osama bin Laden's terrorist organisation, Al Qa'ida destroyed the lives of so many in the World Trade Center. The result of which is that tourism to anywhere other than recognised western world countries is sadly depleted, it hasn't stopped completely, but numbers are down dramatically. When we travelled to Morocco in October 2001 we were shown the same warmth by the local population as we were this time in Egypt. All those involved in the tourism industry were outwardly appreciative that we had the confidence to visit their country during difficult times and made the sincerest of statements that included, please regard this as your second home, or just simply, welcome home. They really meant it rather than the hollow statements issued without any sincerity at all by 'primed up' sales staff at retail outlets in other parts of the world, including our own.

The lack of fellow guests on our Nile cruiser, a five star luxury floating hotel was self evident. On a vessel designed to accommodate 200 passengers in 100 spacious cabins, there were just 40 of us for the whole of the week's cruise from Luxor to Aswan and back. Just a casual glance at an attentive member of the ship's company was enough to see them come to your side and enquire if they could be of service, the crew numbered 25 to serve the 40 guests, a ratio of nearly 2:1. Because there were so few passengers, space to ourselves was freely available, whether it be in the lounge or on the top deck where there were ample wicker chairs, tables and sun shades. The outside of the vessel was washed and polished every day, the en-suite shower room had the towels changed twice daily and fresh bed linen every single day. The polite and attentive crew were paid very little and rely heavily on gratuities given collectively by the guests which were subsequently shared on an equal basis between every single crew member from kitchen porter to helmsman. Despite their low income, these crew members were in fact better off than most of the villagers they'd left at home. They were fed, accommodated, given a uniform which they wore with pride and most importantly, a status. To give passengers a feeling of security and protection, just in case, when the vessel moored up overnight it would be guarded by one or two members of the Egyptian Tourist Police. No one was allowed to enter the boat via the gang plank unless they produced a boarding card, even on embarkation the passengers had to go through a screening device similar to those installed at airports, safety of the passengers was paramount. The police officers, dressed distinctly in white combat uniforms with black berets and carrying AK-47 automatic weapons which were probably older than the users, would occasionally accompany the boat from one mooring stop to another.

They too are paid almost nothing and it gave them the chance to be fed and watered before hitching a ride back to their starting point later that day and take another meal en route. The highlight of the cruise was after we had moored at Aswan where we boarded a 20 foot metal launch and motored up through the cataracts to a Nubian village in the lee of the Aswan dam and backing onto the Libyan desert. The race has been indigenous to the region for 5,000 years and are tall and gracious with an immense sense of pride. Some of their neighbours had to be re-located when the valley was flooded following construction of the dam which created Lake Nasser, the largest man-made lake in the world. We were invited into the home of one family who occupied a 5,000-year-old mud dwelling with a reeded roof and a propane gas cooker on which they boiled water for the delicious hibiscus tea which they served to all visitors.

Although they extended their hospitality to us, we were however invited to buy trinkets that they had made for the tourist to take home, they cost practically nothing and the extra revenue was more than welcomed by the villagers. With no roads serving the village, everything has to come in by boat or across the desert, the ubiquitous Coca-Cola was in evidence as a mark that western world influences can be found in the middle of a desert, but it is the first time I've seen it delivered on the back of a camel, a gloriously grumpy animal called 'Shark' who would look disdainfully down its proud head as if to say, 'Haven't you seen a camel before?' We were not deterred from visiting Arab or Muslim countries, for if terrorists are going to strike they will do it anywhere in the world as has been proven by other recent terrorist attacks, you are not 100% safe anywhere in the world and if common sense is adopted, there is no reason not to travel to these or any other country, providing of course that there is not a warning from the Foreign Office not to travel as it may invalidate any travel insurances.

The End

As our Christmas plans had been so severely disrupted last year because of my relapse, I was determined to make the most of it this year, so we booked up as a family to have two weeks in Funchal, Madiera. We'd been very happy there two years ago, the climate suited me, the hotel was comfortable, the food relatively unadulterated, so we returned for Christmas and New Year 2002. I'd swum in their outside pool on Boxing Day last time which was quite an emotional thing for my wife Julie to witness for the last time I had attempted to swim it was as if a person was hovering above me with a carving knife. Plunging it into my spine every time I surfaced. On this occasion I was able to swim in comparatively little pain and discomfort, I fully intended to repeat the swim if I could. Madeira is an interesting island, very lush and verdant which can be in stark contrast to the sheer sea cliffs that are the highest in Europe. No visit to Funchal could be considered complete unless tea was taken at Reid's Palace Hotel, sitting on their terrace overlooking the bay is something everyone should participate in, we did. An account of Tea at Reid's and a travelogue on Madeira follows.

THE QUINTESSENTIAL ENGLISH TEA AT REID'S PALACE HOTEL, FUNCHAL, MADEIRA

What could be more English than to take tea on the terrace of one of the finest hotels in the world? That experience can be enjoyed in the quintessential Reid's Palace Hotel overlooking Funchal Bay, Madeira. Built in 1887 by the Englishman, William Reid the hotel was designed by a London architect's practice who had recently completed the renowned Shepheard Hotel in Cairo. The hotel boasts a string of influential visitors over its 110 year history, perhaps one of its most illustrious, being Winston

Churchill who would paint the commanding harbour view from the terrace where today afternoon tea can be taken. He was also to be seen with his easel on a viewing balcony 10km away at Camara de la Lobos and painted the frenetic activity of the fishermen as they repaired nets and hauled their brightly painted boats up the pebble beach. Sadly none of Churchill's paintings were presented to Reid's, so monochrome photos of him painting from there have to suffice.

The walls of the hotel are adorned with many paintings, artefacts and photographs. The most interesting are those showing how the early guests arrived at the hotel, not by road, but by steamer which moored off the deep shelving harbour and were disembarked into launches which pulled up to the hotel's own jetty. An elevator would convey them 50 feet or so to the hotel's main entrance. History does not reveal how many guests or their luggage were given a soaking during this process of 'running the gauntlet' of the Atlantic breakers, but during a subsequent refurbishment of the hotel in the pre-war years, the main entrance was changed to the front of the building, which used to be for the staff and deliveries of supplies. The hotel has been part of the 'Leading Hotels of the World' since it was taken over by Orient-Express Hotels Inc. in 1996.

The 'Allotment Garden' Known as Madeira.

Often described as "The Floating Garden", Madeira is a rocky outcrop in the volcanic archipelago standing in the Atlantic Ocean some 500 miles off the Portuguese mainland. It is the largest of the group of islands, consisting of; Porto Santo with its sandy beaches, and the two uninhabited Deserter's Islands, although seal colonies have flourished there due to their inaccessibility.

Madeira is approximately 60km by 25km and has lush vegetation, due to its wet and warm climate which hardly varies from a temperate F° 72. Discovered in 1418 by Portuguese sailors, and named from the Portuguese language, "Madeira", to suit its largest attribute "timber". So dense was the forestation, that it took seven years of clearing and burning to enable the settlers to have sufficient land to support themselves by growing crops.

The terrain in the centre of the island is, surprisingly flat, despite being 1,810 metres above sea level. The vegetation is heather and gorse, on which a few sheep graze. This plateau, Paul Da Serra, is invariably covered in mist and dew gathers in large, flat dew ponds. The island's irrigation system depends upon water from these hills and mountains to provide sufficient supplies to lower parts via water channels known as "Levadas". So important is the maintenance of these water courses, that a government official is employed to monitor the amount of water drawn off from them. Agriculture plays a very important part in the economy, not for its export potential, but to sustain the inhabitants. Some Madeirense are too poor to visit other parts of the island as they have no transport of their own and not all public transport services extend to the farthest extremes of the island. Those who live close to the island's capital, Funchal, are almost exclusively involved in the tourist industry, whether it be as hotel staff, transport, bar workers etc. It is very much a "those who have, and those who have not" island.

There are no large farms on the island, numerous small-holders have terraced their land to grow crops for their own consumption and vital to their existence. They also keep their cattle in small cow sheds, preventing them from roaming free in case one should fall off the terrace and become lame. The sheds used to have thatched roofs, made from the sugar cane that was once grown commercially. The roofs are now clad almost entirely in corrugated iron as it is far less labour intensive. The sheds look like any well used allotment garden shed in England and from the outside give nothing away to say that they house a valuable commodity, a cow, also vital to its owner's existence.

Cows used to be far more numerous on the island, however disease and trading by unscrupulous traders saw the advent of licensing, registration and even supply by the Madeiran government. The land holder must pay a tax each year to keep his animal which cost around 700 Euro, about £500 to purchase. I met a sun and wind tanned small-holder and owner of a cow called 'MALHÁDA' (two coloured), Alfredo Da Costa who at only 52 looked ten to fifteen years older due to the extremely arduos task of keeping his family in provisions from a plot not much larger than an 20 rod allotment garden. Alfredo and his family, live on the northeast coast of the island in the village of Santana, (Saint Anna) renowned for it's "A" framed, thatch roofed houses. There are still examples to be seen, however most are for the benefit of the tourist's camera and have been re-created in a convenient location close to the village centre. However a short walk along some of the village's lanes will let the visitor see some of the original houses, now mostly extended with brick walls and tiled roofs. In addition to requiring extra living accommodation, the more permanent structures are less likely to burn down! Alfredo's brother, Emanuel (79) lives in one such house with his wife and 92 years old mother-in-law. "The cow used to live downstairs under the house" he informed me, I didn't dare ask any further questions.

Sunday 23rd February 2003

I think that my shingles have returned, I've got a rash at the base of my spine. I'll tell the hospital in case it's important.

Friday 28th February 2003

Specialist has given me Aciclovir for shingles, it's not too extensive and should go very shortly.

Tuesday 4th March 2003

Temperature of 38.7, specialist says it's a chest infection and I'm to have antibiotics. Shingles almost gone now.

Tuesday April Fool's Day 2003

We took the chance to fly off to Florida from Gatwick with Continental Airlines, I'd been to Chicago in October last year, but my wife, Julie, had yet to make the pilgrimage across the pond and was a little sceptical about it because we were independent travellers rather than going on an escorted tour with all the arrangements and thinking done for us. Our destination in Florida was Sarasota, there wasn't a direct flight to that airport so a change of planes in New York was required. At least we had the chance to stretch our legs for a while instead of sitting on a plane for 9 or 10 hours. Rather than trying to find our way to the apartment in the dark, we had booked into a motel close to the airport and used the shuttle bus service to get there, we would return to the airport the next day to collect the hire car, which we subsequently named 'Hank'.

We spent two very happy weeks in Sarasota, the people were wonderful, we coped with the excessive amounts of food served in the restaurants by sharing portions. The weather was good in April, not too hot at around the eighties, the wildlife including alligators were interesting and we look forward to returning whenever time and health permits. A travelogue follows.

PETER'S LIVE DIARY SARASOTA, FLORIDA

Tuesday 1st April 2003

Not perhaps the most well chosen date to fly across the Atlantic, some fool or joker might have just declared he's planted a device on the aeroplane delaying or cancelling the flight. However, no such incident was reported, possibly in view of the extra tight precautions at London's Gatwick Airport where everyone was subjected to having their footwear x-rayed to ensure that no device was concealed within. I got away without a check because my boat shoes were so flat and incapable of hiding anything, my wife however had higher shoes with a reinforcing bar to lift the instep, which caused suspicion and needed further inspection. That done we passed through the International Departure gate to board our Continental Airlines, Boeing 777 bound for New York's Newark Liberty airport.

It would appear that Continental value the mature status of their cabin crew with 50% being aged around 50 years of age compared to twenty-somethings of other fleet carriers. The flight was remarkably smooth and comfortable despite flying 'Coach Class'. We left Gatwick on time at 11:50 and landed at Liberty at 13:00 Eastern Standard Time, a flight of just over six hours. We couldn't get immediate flights to Orlando or even the regional airport at Sarasota, so we had a five hour wait at Liberty before our connecting flight to Sarasota-Bradenton International Airport, just 15 minutes from our final destination. The time soon passed once we had had a meal and made good use of Continental's President's Lounge made available to us courtesy of the airline and my friend David. As Liberty is the first point of entry into the USA for many travellers, we had to fill in the necessary immigration forms and queue to go through Passport Control to get our passports stamped, a stub of the immigration form stapled to our passports which would be removed when leaving the country, that way the authorities know (theoretically) how many non nationals are in the country, logistically it would be a nightmare to even start to establish how many. If a barcode system were incorporated into the stub it would be easier because a scanner would record the numbers, still it's not up to me to tell George W. Bush how to run his country!

Sarasota-Bradenton was a much larger airport than I expected, modern and clean and at 21:00 local time, was almost empty. We had arranged to collect a car from Alamo-National car hire, but decided that we would overnight in a hotel and collect the car in the daylight as it was our first venture into the American road system. The first language barrier was encountered here when I asked the sales clerk where the courtesy telephones were for the hotel's shuttle bus. "Right over there by the kiosk" came the answer. Now we Brits regard a kiosk as a cabin, booth, or even a shop, their kiosk was what we would call a counter or console. "Sorry I can't see it" I exclaimed, then the American version of a female John Cleese cut in, "There, there, over there!" in an almost irritated tone giving credence to the saying that we are two countries separated by a common language!

I duly phone the Holiday Inn and arrange transport to the hotel and walk out of the airport to the pick up point, where a minibus awaits. We get in and drive to the Hilton hotel together with all the flight crew, "Are you staying here?" the driver asks and it's then I realise that we are at the wrong hotel. "I thought we were going to the Holiday Inn as well" I mumble and as quick as a flash he offers to drive us to our chosen hotel some 3 miles away. I give him an unexpected tip of a couple of dollars to buy a coffee and we arrive at the Holiday Inn where I have some explaining to do. "I rang for a minibus collection and got on the wrong bus" I announce expecting another tirade of officialdom. "No problem," comes the reply and our luggage is carried to the first floor of the 1950's built two storey hotel which was once a motel. "Why don't they pull this place down and build a modern hotel?" I ask innocently. "This is one of the oldest buildings in Sarasota" I am indignantly informed. "They've spent millions on it!" Where and how is one of the all time mysteries as the door has gaps around it wide enough to let in most bugs and creepy-crawlies, the shower fails to yield even warm water and there's no lift. Having said that; the staff were polite to the nth. degree and the view from the breakfast room across the marina was one which would see me re-visit just for the atmosphere alone.

Wednesday 2nd April 2003

The minibus we should have ridden in last night has now taken us back to the airport to collect our rental car. We are asked if we want an upgrade (for an extra charge) and we decide that even their compact cars are larger than our Punto back home and settle for the Chevrolet Cavalier that was originally assigned to us. "It's in the lot opposite," we are informed. We step outside and all a person can see in front of them, are rental cars in parking lots! Eventually we find 'Hank' the hire car, familiarise ourselves with the controls for the air-con and the steering wheel being on the wrong side and progress at a snail's pace out on to the Tamiami Trail (Interstate Highway 41) in search of the University Parkway and our eventual home for two weeks in an apartment at the other end of the freeway. Miracle upon miracle, we find it without getting lost thanks to the idiot proof instructions gleaned from other members of the family who have stayed there and proceed to disgorge our possessions from Hank. The weather is wonderful, 80° and no humidity, I could get used to this. One of the first things we do after unpacking is to have that hot shower which evaded us at Holiday Inn Heritage Motel. I can't get the water to come out of the tap (faucet), I can't even turn the blessed thing on. The instructions were, "In case of ANY problems with the apartment, phone the house sitter for advice", so I phone and pretend to be an incapable English Snow-Bird who doesn't know how to operate the taps. I need not have pretended, because she knew I was exactly what I said I was, an incapable English person inarticulate in the operation of American taps. "I have to visit nearby," we are told, "I'll call in," which an hour later she does. A charming lady who looks after the apartment when it's not occupied and whose husband does the odd jobs around the place. I am relieved to know that I wasn't being stupid, the washer, or cartridge as they call them, is in need of replacement which after a couple of days is attended to.

We have no food in the house and need to stock up, reference is made to the idiot proof instructions again and we take Hank off to the supermarket at Sarasota Crossings. We armed ourselves with a cool-box from the apartment as in this heat any frozen food would have started to defrost by the time we were home. We decide to eat first so that we can make a dash for home afterwards while the food is still reasonably fresh. 'Wings and Weenies' was opposite the car parking bay and we enter and share a plateful of chicken wings, curly fries and a choice of dressing. "What dressing do you want, blue cheese or ranch?" "What's ranch?" we enquire and rather than the waitress explaining to stupid English people, gives us both anyway. It turns out to be garlic and herb, why don't they just say so? The food is excellent, as it is all over Florida and cheap. The next brave step is to explore the 'Publix Supermarket'.

What a choice! I don't usually go into supermarkets in this country, but this place had a deli to die for, we stock up with all the essentials, gin, Martini, olives, oh and some other food stuff as well. Just like Continental Airlines, Publix seems to favour the mature worker. Our packer was Amos and I inanely comment that Andy must be at the next check-out. I get a look that says, "Stupid English Snow-Bird" (those who migrate to warmer climes during the English winter). "No Andy hasn't finished his paper round yet" I am informed, I don't know who was having the greatest laugh out of this, him or me!

We push our trolley to the car park and look for a bay in which to leave it, "Just leave it on the side and we'll collect it" I am politely informed and then try to open the boot (trunk) of a gold coloured Cavalier which turned out not to be our car. Luckily the car had no alarm system and we were not observed. It doesn't make life any easier for the stupid Brits when American cars don't have licence plates on the front of the vehicle and with no nodding dogs or fluffy dice in the window, how on earth are you supposed to recognise which is your car? We eventually find our car and make our way gingerly out onto the service road where a man of around 35 was carrying a box of liquor from the off licence. I watch him closely because there's not much of his eyes visible over the top of the box, but he keeps on coming, right in front of the car and I'm forced to come to an abrupt stop. Another tirade follows when I'm informed that "It's state law, cars give way to pedestrians!" I wish someone at Alamo-National had thought to mention that when we collected the car, it would have saved us from a potentially difficult situation.

After exploring our immediate environs, we settle down to an aperitif and microwave a box of something we bought earlier. By now the effect of being awake for twenty hours the day earlier catches up with us and we hit they hay at 20:30 local time and sleep very soundly.

Thursday 3rd April 2003

The weather upon waking was another glorious day, going to be 83° according to Down Town local radio 'The Dove' serving Sarasota and Bradenton with a reminder that we shouldn't forget to call into Arnie's window and door showroom if we want to add 15% value to our apartment. Seeing it isn't ours anyway, we ignore the advise and concentrate on reading the back of American cereal packets just in case they are any more interesting than our own, they weren't, they put over the message that we should recycle our rubbish and are pleased to note that a recycling bin is within 200 yards of where we're staying. That piece of information was not printed on the packet or relayed to us over 'The Dove's ' airways, we found it on our way to the apartment's swimming pool which has to be checked daily to ensure that none of the errant alligators had mistakenly found their way in there rather than the adjacent lagoon.

Time to explore Sarasota itself. Our idiot proof notes tell us exactly which road to take but we still manage to get lost when the road we were following changed its name and didn't advise us it was about to do that. We wait at a red traffic light and get hooted at for not going against it. You are allowed to turn right at a junction when the light is against you if there are no cars, we proceed with the utmost caution as the thought of having to fill in American insurance claim forms is a daunting prospect. We park in a car park close to the library and try to work out where to slot the dollar bill for our parking fee. The slot which issues the receipt is the exact size to take a dollar bill, but doesn't, it's a coin-operated meter pure and simple. We have no coins, it is at that point that a lady police officer sees a stupid English person and comes over with a handful of coins for me to feed the meter, she would take no payment in return, "what a nice person" I thought, and she was. Selby Library is vast, new and a pleasure to be in compared to English, "Don't you dare talk in here" libraries. We want to email a relative and go to the counter to meet yet another mature volunteer who allows us one hours free access to a computer. He gives us another set of idiot proof instructions how to re-trace our steps to the apartment without getting lost, "I live there too so I know the best route", he said. On the development where the apartment is situated, stands a small shopping area in which there is a deli from where food can be pre-ordered and taken back to the apartment to be consumed at leisure. We eat our supper to the sounds of an American type crow, known as a Greckle, continuously saying "Eh Oh." I didn't know that the Tellytubbies had found their way over to Florida. We call it a day at 20:30 again and settle down for yet another deep sleep in a king size bed that almost needs another set of idiot proof instructions with directions to find your way out of it.

Friday 4th April 2003

A busy day ahead of us, we breakfast, study the road map and head off up the Interstate Highway number 75 past the Tampa turn off to the regional airfield of Lakeland-Linder where there is the annual Sun n' Fun Fly In. The journey of approximately 120 miles takes us an hour and three quarters as we carefully pick our way through unfamiliar territory, road works and streams of well driven lorries, camper vans and car loads of excited children whose final destination is to see Mickey (who ever he is?). What an array of aircraft! I've never seen so many war birds in one place outside the film of Pearl Harbour. There was a mock bombing run with a little man setting off cans of Kerosene which resulted in magnificent black smoke rings just hanging in the still spring air and 87° temperature. We take lunch courtesy of the Press Tent and I enjoy my first taste of 'Pork n' Beans' and can't get enough of it. I'm asked if I want a cobbler but uncertain if there was an on-site shoe repairer or what, I enquire as to its origins and presented with a wonderful fruit compote, why don't they call it so, these Americans do speak strangely! I've worn myself and my wife ragged, running around looking at this, looking at that, going in here, there and everywhere, eventually I come to my senses and get a golf cart to take us back to the car park before we both expire, not from the heat but the physical endurance of trying to see everything there was to see, it was impossible!

We were very confused by the scenery en route to Lakeland. The buildings looked a little Moroccan, albeit a modern shopping complex, trees and the river reminded us of a trip down the Nile and the temperature was identical to both countries. We had to keep reminding ourselves that we were in Florida. Having left the air show reasonably early to avoid the mass exodus, we were home by 17:00 just in time to go to 'our' deli for essential supplies of milk, papers and doughnuts and tell them how good their Shepherd's Pie was, despite the fact that it was beef. Following this we sat on the porch and enjoyed a 'sharpener' before dinner, retiring no later than we have all week so far, lights out at 21:00 exhausted.

Saturday 5th April 2003

We take a stroll from the apartment along a track that skirts a golf course, only to be intercepted by a brace of men in a golf cart stating that, "People have right of way over bicycles along here, but a golf cart has right of way over everything except cars, and you won't find one on this track!" Not being certain if we have transgressed another state law, we beat a hasty retreat and find ourselves a footpath over which we have definite right of way to the local shopping area. We avail ourselves of the bottomless coffee pot at the deli, a doughnut and bought an English newspaper printed in Florida. We take Hank for a drive into Sarasota and park alongside the waterfront, no meters this time so no nice lady police officers to assist us. At the south east end of the causeway, dotted with sculptures and other artistic devises, is the Marie Selby Botanical Garden, an oasis of calm against the relentless hum of traffic on the Tamiami Trail (U.S. 41) that passes within 100 yards at one point. It is an important facility for training botanists and boasts a Koi carp pond, mangrove swamp, board walk and a canopy walk enabling the visitor to get a bird's eye view of the rich in species, and particularly lush foliage.

The entrance fee is $10.00 and worth every cent (or penny as they quaintly refer to them over there). There is a particularly favourite watering hole of ours on the bay front, Marina Jack's where we are often to be found sipping cool soft drinks or sharing one of their meals, a meal each is too much for us, although most Americans seem to manage it, if they can't they ask for a doggy bag and finish it later. The enclosed terrace has wonderful views across the harbour and out into the bay, a boater's paradise, but sadly I don't have a boat. Having had a previously good record of finding our way back home, we relax our guard and get lost, hopelessly lost. A man washing his car detects the bewildered look of a lost sole and deduces it must come from a Brit. "What part of England are you from?" we are asked. It's easier to say Brighton on the seaside as it's almost as famous, or infamous as London. "I lived on a boat in Brighton Marina for eight years and was born in Croydon," we were told. He gave us instructions how to get home, which at the time sounded implausible, we try and follow them but find ourselves going past the end of his road again some 20 minutes later. The problem is that there are roads either end of town with the same name, but don't connect in the middle, perhaps one day the master plan would be to link them up, but at present they don't and it confuses the already bewildered English tourist. The temperature is still in the low 80's and very, very pleasant, it's a warmth that you can easily get used to and makes a damp English springtime a distant memory.

Sunday 6th April 2003

Today is the day that the Floridians put their clocks back by one hour, back in England we did it last week, but now that the rest of the civilised world are copying our time keeping habits you would have thought that we could all change the clocks on the same day, but no! We never really caught up with the difference between Eastern Standard Time and Pacific Time anyway, so to be an hour adrift from British Summer Time didn't seem to matter because we were five hours ahead of them already, or was that six hours before they altered their clocks? Now, there are those who will no doubt correct me on this, but I observed that the water from the bath goes down the plughole anti-clockwise compared to clockwise over here. I wasn't aware of having crossed the Equator, but it was a personal observation and one on which I am prepared to be corrected. I wasn't really bored over there, I just noticed it one day, as you do and made a note of it!

The Brazilian Grand Prix is being run today, so when we return to Marina Jack's for lunch of chicken wrap, I enquire if anyone knows the result. I might just have easily been asking who won the Martian Marble Levitating competition. "We don't follow it over here" I was informed by the twenty-something year old restaurant manager, "but I'll find out for you", which he did bless him. He was very interested to learn about the culture of young English college students. "Do they all fly off to the sun during the Easter break as ours do, or what?" I replied that most college kids take part-time work during the holiday and would only have a day out by the seaside if the weather permitted, i.e. wasn't snowing during Easter. This he thought hilarious. We saw no skinheads, lager louts and saw only respect amongst the younger population for their contemporaries. "I'm sorry sir," one 18 yr old said as he inadvertently stepped into my path whilst I was walking, it may have been different if I was driving as he may have quoted the state law at me, issued a writ or immediately phoned his lawyer. We didn't see any litter either, no Big Mac cartons, fag ends, chewing gum, White Lightning cider cans, nothing. They must impose a hefty on the spot fine if anyone is caught being a litter bug and we didn't see one example of graffiti either, what a difference from anywhere in England or the continent even. Along the walkway by the side of Harbour Park is a small enclave of Englishness, firstly a Punch and Judy Man has set up camp there and entertains the bewildered American kids with strings of sausages, crocodiles and 'iffy' looking policemen all talking in an even more 'iffy' accent. Some children were puzzled, some were crying, I'm not surprised at either. Adjacent to his stand is O'Leary's Bar at which a 50-year-old, long haired guitarist is playing all time American classics to a fairly disinterested audience. He gets fed and watered and the occasional dollar bill, but has a wonderful all year round tan and an easy lifestyle and sadly doesn't need an assistant. O'Leary has an ice cream cabinet in his bar which catches our attention. Two wrapped confections are bought and I proffer four one dollar bills and enquire if it's enough? The reply comes in a thick West Midlands accent which states that "If I take just four dollars from you, I can't afford the airfare home". As he's been there for eight years anyway, his argument didn't seem to hold much water. He came on holiday from Birmingham one spring and just didn't want to go home. "I thought about it, Birmingham or Florida? No contest!"

Although still warm at 80+°, the weather is becoming a little overcast, no longer do we see the clear cobalt blue skies that we enjoyed earlier in the week. It may possibly rain, they do need it so badly in Florida as there has been a drought for the last two years and even the Everglades are drying up, tonight might change their fortunes.

Monday 7th April 2003

No it didn't rain and today looks like being another scorcher. The Selby Library is revisited today as we want to check for emails from home, it's not that we can't bear to be parted from them, it's just that it's nice to keep in touch and it's quicker (and cheaper) than sending a post-card (which we eventually do anyway!). We have lunch and notice a group of twenty or so ladies of indeterminate age all sporting red hats and most wearing purple dresses, there was one man amongst them wearing a purple shirt, I think he may have been the husband of one of the ladies as officially he shouldn't be a member, even though they had no rules. I enquire as to the reason for so many similarly dressed women and was informed that the 'Red Hat Club' meets at different locations in Florida every month, there are no rules and no dues, it's just a reason for ladies to have a jolly good day out. There was however one rebel amongst the group, she defied convention and wore a red dress and purple hat, but as there's no rules, who cares?

Should this organisation cross the pond, I would be one of the first to add my name to its list of members and follow the dictate within the following passage which is from a slightly amended version of a poem by Jenny Joseph to whom apologies are sent.

A Warning

When I am an old man I shall wear purple

With a red hat which doesn't go and doesn't suit me,

And I shall spend my pension on brandy and summer gloves

And satin shirts, and say we've no money for butter.

I shall sit down on the pavement when I'm tired

And gobble up samples in shops and press alarm bells

And run my stick along public railings

And make up for the sobriety of my youth

I shall go out in my slippers in the rain

And pick flowers in others people's gardens

And learn to spit.

You can wear terrible shirts and grow more fat

And eat three pounds of sausages at a go

Or only bread and pickle for a week

And hoard pens and pencils and beer-mats and things in boxes.

But we must have clothes that keep us dry
And pay our rent and not swear in the street
And set a good example to our children
We must have friends to dinner and read the papers.

But maybe I ought to practice a little now?
So people who know me are not too shocked and surprised
When suddenly I am old and start to wear purple!
End.

It's supermarket sweep time again, we return to Publix and are instantly recognised by the checkout lady, we really must stick out like sore thumbs. On our return to our base camp we disgorge the shopping and head for the complexes swimming pool. Good news, still no 'gators in it. During these times of drought, it is not implausible for them to nuisance themselves in private pools, I'd do the same! There's no one else in the water and at first the water seems cold until I get used to it and then I don't want to get out. The air temperature is 83° again and still no real sign of rain.

Tuesday 8th April 2003

There's a 30% chance of rain today, although you wouldn't think it if you looked outside at the clear blue sky devoid of any cloud, but it may change, The Dove says so anyway. Time to explore more of the area, so we drive into Sarasota, along Bay Front Road and across the Siesta Key Bridge, a new one is being built adjacent to it, high enough to facilitate a yacht with its mast up, at present passage is restricted. We pull into a car park just over the bridge for a photo shoot opportunity and watch pelicans diving for their food. Some however were 'street wise' and waited by the side of the quay for fishermen to empty their catch of shrimp into a bucket, some of which always lands on the floor where the fish are quickly devoured by the waiting birds. Access to the beach is easy, there are several free car parks that all look the same. Some kind person has numbered them to avoid the visitor trudging miles in the heat trying to locate their car. There's still no sign of rain and if anything, the day is becoming hotter with each passing hour. I wanted to call upon the manager of a beachside resort hotel who had been kind enough to offer complementary accommodation over the Christmas period in 2001, however circumstances dictated that we couldn't take her up on the offer so I thought it would be nice to thank her in person, she was having a day off! I made no promises to return as we are fairly restricted for time and don't want to miss out on other 'sightseeing' attractions. Back home on the development where our temporary home is located, we take advantage of the numerous cycle tracks. First however, I had to extricate the bikes from the cupboard, attach wheels, adjust saddles, pump up tyres etc. I was almost too tired to ride the bike after all that! However ride we did in glorious sunshine and still no sign of the much needed rain. I sit on the back porch, gin and tonic in hand and write postcards pretending to miss people back home, I suppose I do really, it's just that this place is so idyllic.

Wednesday 9th April 2003

Still a promise of rain, skies are now more than just overcast and reports of snow in New York with temperatures of minus 2°, here the temperature has dropped to around 66°, I can live with that. Before the rain does come, we walk to the village shops and deli and settle down to a large mug of coffee and a doughnut. A couple we met, Marilyn and Edwin are keen to show us two alligators that are currently occupying the lagoon adjacent to the stores. The 'gators are just cruising up and down looking for an excuse to venture out of the water and take someone's leg off, that is if they can be bothered and by the look of them, they can't!

Excitement over, we head off on the U.S. 41 to the Ringling Museum, a magnificent edifice built by John and Mabel Ringling (of Ringling Bros. Circus fame) in 1926, sadly Mabel was only there for three years until she died but what she achieved with an array of interior designers and builders, is impressive. The whole site, was until its construction, a desolate piece of real estate out on the very edge of civilisation with only a dirt track lane giving any access to the town, now there's a three lane highway going in three directions from it. The style of architecture is very Italianate, although a bit of Gothic creeps in and the interior of Cà d'Zan (John's House) shows a French connection and the general mixture of 'Magpie' culture, 'If it's shiny, I want it', a typical trait of 'new money'. It is however impressive that so much was achieved in such a short time and the state must be appreciative of John Ringling when he bequeathed it upon his death in 1936. I couldn't find the 'Secret Garden' (must be very well hidden) and didn't have time to visit the circus museum, I'll leave that until next time, for as sure as eggs is eggs, there'll be another time. We get back to base camp at 16:30 and it starts to rain, the skies are heavy with thunder clouds and the temperature has dropped to 73° making it feel as if a good old fashioned storm is about to break, but it doesn't, it just continues to rain lightly.

Thursday 10th April 2003

The Dove still says there's a high possibility of rain today, the wind has got up and it no longer looks or feels as though we're in the Sunshine State of Florida. Not much point in going too far afield today, so we walk to the post box to send off the last of the postcards. American boxes, or those in Sarasota anyway are designed around the all important motor car. They are at the correct height to pop in a letter whilst still in your car and they all face the pavement edge to make it even easier for those who do not, or cannot get out of the car. In England, the Post Office site them away from the curb, have the slot facing away from the road and place the opening at a height that makes it impossible to access unless you are over six foot six tall and always drive an open top car, or ride on a bicycle. Duty done, we continue our walk, yes we walked to the post box and received strange looks from motorists attending to their mail from the comfort of their cars, to the deli for coffee and cheesecake Danish pastries, they sound a bit weird but taste divine.

We stock up on milk and the Daily Mail and return to the apartment, only to find we have nothing for lunch so walk back to the deli and share a chicken wrap with some salad and fries, delicious. I wanted to video the alligators in the pond, but they too were out to lunch so I'll just have to carry the camera around with me wherever I go and look like a tourist not a resident until they do show up. In the afternoon we go to Selby Library in the middle of Sarasota to send and check emails, another grey haired volunteer is polite to us, talks to us not through us and allows us access to a PC. Having passed a golf club en route to the library which must have had around sixty golf carts parked outside, I have re-christened this part of Florida from 'The Gold Coast State', to 'The Golf Cart State'. "Can I hire one for a day?" I enquire, "No but give me eighteen hundred dollars and it's yours!" came the reply. If petrol, sorry, gas, wasn't so cheap, a golf cart might have been a good investment to zoom about in, although they only look as if they're going fast when you're walking, I expect you'd soon get fed up with their 10 mph top speed. I didn't buy one, I filled Hank up with gas for the equivalent of £10.00 instead.

Friday 11th April 2003

Because our tickets home on the airline were 'stand by', I thought I'd check with airport to see if there was a likelihood of seats or not. Although it was a full flight, we were told that there was a good chance of getting home, pity really I was just beginning to get used to the Floridian way of life. En route back from the airport and opposite the Ringling Museum is the Sarasota Classic Car Museum. There's a pink Cadillac on the roof and outside rests a couple of ageing autos, not rusting as it is a good climate for keeping a car for three decades. Inside we are treated to antique advertising posters, old slot machines and an array of vintage 'stuff' not strictly connected to auto-memorabilia, but interesting all the same. There are model 'T' Fords, the Beatles Beetle Cabriolet, John Lennon's Mercedes convertible and a Ford Anglia, E93A, right hand drive and almost identical with my first car. You know when you're getting old because the things you used every day are museum pieces and kids say "Gee Mom, look at that crazy old car!" Even cameras that I've got stashed away somewhere are exhibited here, I'm so taken aback that I forget to turn off the record button on the cam-corder and have several feet on film of very nicely brick tiled flooring to show people, they'll be impressed. We sit and recuperate with an ice cream and soda-pop and meet an octogenarian who had no where to go all day except hang around ice cream bars and parking lots. No don't feel sorry for him, he owned two apartments and has moved out of his to earn more rent. "I'm thinking of buying a third" he said gleefully and probably will settle down for the night at the same 'Heritage Centre Motel' that we spent our first night in when I suggested to the manager that it ought to be pulled down and rebuilt up to modern standards.

On our return to base camp, I wrestle with getting the bike out of the porch cupboard again and once again take to the cycle tracks with camera slung over my shoulder in case I bump into Mr & Mrs 'Gator, but it's the breeding season and they'll be too busy doing what 'gators do, to pose for a 'Limey' visitor. Previously, I'd espied a 'Rack o' Ribs Shack' offering 2lbs of ribs for $10.00. I can't resist ribs, so we pick up our pre-ordered dinner and spot out of the corner of our eye a chiller counter with cheesecake in, I can't resist cheesecake either, so home we go laden down with as many bags as you normally collect from a Chinese take-away establishment. The temperature is still a chillier 67° but 'the Dove' promises that the weather will improve by the weekend, let's hope so.

Saturday 12th April 2003

It's sunny and warm again and back to typical Floridian weather thank goodness, so we venture out again to places we have yet to visit. First however, I must just snatch a chance glimpse of a 'gator in the lagoon. I go armed with digital and video cameras and lo and behold, there he is. I say he but I have no way of knowing if it's a he or a she and no particular desire to find out, a 'gator's a 'gator to all but another 'gator which I ain't! He or she is not particularly active, in fact it just sits there in the mud shallows waiting to cause trouble. Looking at it now it seems incapable of causing any trouble but don't be deceived, what did Kermit's nephew, Robin say? "Never smile at a crocodile, don't be taken in by his cheerful grin" etc. I know that was about a crocodile and this was an alligator, but the principle's the same. On the same lagoon, there is an assembly of retired gentlemen (I use the term guardedly) who race Marblehead boats (model yachts to the uninitiated). Not only do they have to manoeuvre around buoys, but have to miss the 'gators in case one of them takes a bite out of his transom. Retired, they are, gentlemen they may not always be, "Water, water!" one will cry, "No I'm mast abeam!" comes the retort. "You've got to do a 360°" shouts the adjudicator, the real thing is not as aggressive as these guys make it out to be. Still if they weren't here racing yachts they'd be at Publix packing for Brits who make inane comments.

We lunch at Marina Jack's on some delicious seafood something or other and head off across the bridge to St. Armand's Circle. A good 50% of all the white lining in Florida must be at the Circle. Bearing in mind that pedestrians have right of way over everything except golf carts, of which there are none in the Circle, motorists have to tip-toe over the multitude of painted pedestrian crossings. It doesn't end with crossings, there are parking bays, no parking areas, no waiting areas and unloading bays, not unnaturally, the traffic moves very slowly, it doesn't worry us as we're driving so slowly anyway to avoid hitting anything at all. I got particularly worried when I saw a sign stating "Quiet area, Manatees" and then was relieved to see it was in the adjacent bayou.

I take a photo of what I believe to be St. Armand holding a sword, it looked impressive until I got nearer and realised I'd photographed the back of it and the sword turned out to be a steel reinforcing rod, stupid Brits coming over here like Japanese tourists with their snap happy attitude, you hear them mumble under their breathe, except you don't because they are far too polite. I then commit the most sinful thing you can ever do in St. Armand's Circle, I go into an ice cream parlour (where there are more flavours than you can shake a stick at) and ask for a pre-wrapped 'Butter-Finger' or the equivalent. The owner could hardly believe his ears, "You want what?" came the incredulous reply. "You see I have a dietary problem and can only eat pre-wrapped" I lamely state and leave before I get a scoop of his finest pistachio and guava ice cream missile hurtled at the back of my neck. I really needed an ice cream as the temperature has risen to 78° and needed liquid to prevent dehydration, so it's back to Marina Jack's for a long, cool cranberry juice, "Oh, and light on the ice, eh!"

Sunday 13th April 2003

Today is the day of the London Marathon and I'm anxious to learn if Paula Radcliffe was successful in winning for her second consecutive year, however in view of the trouble I caused when asking about the Grand Prix, I decide to wait until I get home. I still don't know who won!

The last few supplies we need before leaving base camp are picked up from Publix, haven't tried Winn-Dixie yet, we'll leave that pleasure for when we return to Florida. At the risk seeming repetitive, we decide to take lunch at, yes you've guessed it, Marina Jack's. Main reason being that we were about to take the boat trip around Sarasota bay and the restaurant is two minutes from the dock. Le Barge is an all metal snub nosed 60' long metal work horse that has two unusual features. Firstly, it has four palm trees growing out of its superstructure, and secondly an indoor aquarium which once we set sail, sees the occupants swished about as if they were in a tidal race. Do fish get seasick I wonder?

The two hour trip was excellent value at $15.00 a throw and takes you to places that wouldn't be accessible by any other means of transport, like outside the house belonging to Jerry Springer and underneath the Siesta Key bridge with its see through metal decking to give you a manatee eye view of eight wheeled trucks and fire tenders. There's still time to call into the Selby Public Library to check for emails from home and we're back at base camp in time to catch the last of the afternoon's warming sunshine and take a bike ride around the area. I've no video camera with me so it's almost a certainty that I'll see an alligator, which I did. They're playing hide and seek with me.

Monday 14th April 2003

We don't want to leave Sarasota, but we have a plane to catch. It isn't until tomorrow, but I don't want to be sitting for a couple of hours in a car and then another ten hours on an aeroplane. We've packed up the apartment, put the rubbish out, put our belongings in Hank, by 11:00 we're on the road again. Have I got enough petrol to get me to Orlando I wonder? I don't really want to fill up again seeing that Hank gets dropped off the next day, I estimate that unless we get lost, we've enough for the journey.

With a lunch stop just off the Interstate Highway 75 and a two mile detour to get back on it, petrol's a close thing. Deciding to see exactly where the airport is and finding a hotel close by takes even more petrol but we've seemingly not used as much on the freeway as we would have done around town, so all's well. The Hilton Hotel was within two miles of the terminal building and we decide to overnight there. It has a swimming pool and a fitness suite, I chose the former, leaving the latter to those who know how to use it properly, it's been a long time since I did repetitions and don't want to 'bust a gut' on my last day.

AJ, the hotel's minibus driver is outside the front of the hotel with nothing better to do than kick the tyres and adjust the driving mirror so I approach him for 'idiot proof' instructions on how to (a) find the terminal and (b) where to drop Hank off. "I'll take you there now" he offers and we have to tell him that we're not due to fly out until tomorrow. "No matter. Let's go see anyway!" so we pile in and head off to the airport. "Hold on" I exclaim, "if we're going there now and I don't need the car tomorrow, can we drop it off now?" "Sure thing" states AJ as we return to the hotel and pick up Hank and follow AJ back to the airport. He points us to the ramp where Alamo's car return area is and states that he'll meet us at Bus Bay 18 in 15 minutes. The car return agents are all geared up to make things easy for the driver and convenient for themselves. The young man swiped the bar code on the licence holder with a hand held device and immediately he gets a print out to say that all dues have been paid, the return is within the rental period. With that all done he bids us good bye and moves onto the next car in the line. Such efficiency, considering the car was picked up in Sarasota and dropped off in Orlando. AJ is as good as his word and meets us in bay 18 to take us back to the Hilton. He's just picked up a flight crew returning to Orlando and heading for the same hotel. Jim Jeter, a captain, sits opposite me and notices me reading his name badge. "Great name for a jet pilot eh?" he states, "Jim, you mean?" I retort, I'm not sure he understood the British sense of humour and he was glad to strike up a conversation with his colleagues. Although the Hilton Hotel has a breakfast room, it doesn't have a dining room, so we are forced to eat out that evening. We didn't have to go far, for at the bottom of the hotel's car park is a grey-painted hillbilly type shack complete with porch, verandah and is constructed of what we know in England, as 'ship lap' boarding. This establishment is called 'Hooters' and as we step inside and are immediately greeted by up to a dozen scantily dressed teenage girls with orange hot pants and breasts squeezed into white tee shirts with 'Hooters' emblazoned across their chests, I wondered if "hooters" was a euphemism for a specific part of their anatomy. Not wishing to be regarded as a 'dirty old man', I keep my thoughts (and my hands) to myself. My wife observes that apart from her, there is only one other female customer in the place, I can't think why. The place is seething with men brandishing 'six packs', 'beer bellies', there are travelling salesmen, forty-somethings and just about every other type of male that you can imagine, it's obviously very popular. We order a steak sandwich to share and a plate of curly fries. The menu card states that they are designed by a computer and cooked by a moron, they were however delicious, as was every meal we ate in Florida. I had a budget of just $20.00 as neither of us had any more dollar bills, only dollar travellers' cheques. Our waitress, whom I obviously reminded of her grey haired uncle, was kindly towards me and totted (perhaps I shouldn't use the word 'totty' in this context) up the order and said their would be some left over as she hadn't charged me for the soft drinks. It would sound unfair if I said that she could see her tip being eroded by the continuing order, but she really, really was a nice girl and got every cent left over of the $20.00 bill as a tip. She even sat with us and conversed, young people don't do that in England. She thought that we "spoke real cute" and would like to visit England. She's training to be a lawyer so undoubtedly once she's qualified, she'll be able to fly over first class whenever she feels like it!

Tuesday 15th April 2003

In the morning we breakfast in the hotel's light and spacious dining room and I try out an American cooked breakfast. The hash browns are in fact a mound of shredded potato, lightly fried rather than the coated, triangular and 'E' number coloured variety we're used to at home. My eggs were ordered 'sunny side up', "Yep, they'll be just looking back at you," I am informed by our unisex hairdresser lookalike from back home. I enjoyed the 'fry up' considerably.

As we weren't flying out until 14:00, we had time to walk around our immediate environs. There's a lake with a fountain, ducks and still no litter. We haven't seen ANY litter in Florida. I know that at the Walt Disney resorts there are street sweepers who brush the litter down gaps in the pavement to be bagged up by an army of underground workers, but I didn't think the same system was used throughout every street in every town in Florida, George W's little brother Jeb is doing a fine job of keeping the state a good place to live in, and I wouldn't mind doing just that! I don't know how much estate agents charge their clients in Florida when selling a property, but going by the size of the head quarters of the American Society of Realtors, it must be a huge fee. The building was positively palatial with an appointment needed just to walk past it, well it gave that impression anyway.

AJ wasn't on duty today, so Eric took us in his red minibus to the airport terminal. Eric could well have been a Viking, tall, blonde and immensely strong. This he demonstrated by picking up both our suitcases (which the airline had already deemed to be HEAVY) as if they were empty briefcases. He dropped us at the correct terminal and although there are only two, A & B which connect under a huge atrium inside, they are 200 yards apart within the building, which according to Eric would have caused us considerable grief if we had gone to the wrong gate. We're checked in and still have time to grab a quick bite before we fly out to New York's Liberty. There's no catering on the flight, so we have lunch in the terminal. However, the only place 'airside' was a Burger King, apart from a sandwich bar which was specializing in 'Mashed Hog' baps, we settle for a BK. 50% of the customers were Continental flight crews who were provisioning themselves for their respective flights, particularly as there wasn't any food being served en route. Either that, or there was in flight catering and they had decided that a BK was better alternative. Here again, American efficiency was seen to exist in the form of the manager patrolling the queue asking customers what their order would be and speaking on her 'walkie-talkie' to pre-order it for them. The only queue was at the pay desk, so the piping hot food soon became cold anyway.

We leave on time and arrive at Liberty with a couple of hours to waste, so the President's Lounge of Continental Airlines was put to good use again. The Boeing 777 was on the apron close to us and boarding commenced on time for our flight back to London's Gatwick airport. As you would hope for, it was an uneventful flight, with two meals served during the six and a half hour journey during which we saw the dawn break.

Wednesday 16th April 2003

Arriving ahead of schedule at 06:15, we touch down at Gatwick and are almost 'hustled' through passport control and baggage reclaim. Within half an hour of landing we were heading for a restaurant that served cooked breakfasts. Sadly they weren't as good as their American counterparts, but it was better than nothing, just! The 08:25 train was due at platform 5 bound for Shoreham by Sea in 10 minutes time, so we tip a porter to lug our suitcases down the stairs and that's it, our glorious two weeks' holiday was over. Florida is certainly a state we will revisit at some time, but as there are goodness knows how many destinations to visit, it may not be again this year. Let the good times roll.

Friday 18th April 2003

I feel a bit 'coldy' today and have a temperature of 38.2°, rang the hospital who say come in and pack a bag in case. My temperature is now 39.3° so I'll have to be admitted. It's also the second year running that I'm in hospital on our wedding anniversary!.

I have a very poor record for being on hand, or at home to celebrate significant family events. I'm usually in hospital rather than at birthday parties, weddings or blessings, it wasn't my fault I told my disappointed wife/daughter/son-in-law, I'd see if I could do any better for next year's celebrations.

Sunday 20th April 2003

Temperature is now down to 37.5° and I'm to be allowed home. There was a family wedding in Norwich the following Saturday, so I needed to feel well enough to travel, which this time I did. We stayed at a hotel close to the city centre and Julie ate something at dinner which disagreed with her very badly indeed. A doctor was rung for by the hotel at 02:00 who diagnosed food poisoning. The hotel could not do enough for us and wouldn't allow us to pay on leaving, as if that wasn't enough, we were invited back for a 'free' weekend whenever we wanted, which we accepted for September of that year for another family occasion. The wedding reception was also held at the same hotel, so the level of catering, which was already high, was exceptionally good in every respect, just in case!

Saturday 3rd May 2003

Sad news, Brian, one of our 'cancer club' members died today in a hospice in Worthing, he or I often had to vacate a cubicle on Erringham Ward if the other was more poorly and needed the isolation of a private room.

His subsequent funeral was a very emotional affair and attended by some of the nurses we all knew from the day ward, my eyes were red from weeping.

Friday 16th May 2003

We travelled up to Rickmansworth to a narrow boat festival where my grandfather's boats Arcturus *and* Sirius *were taking part in the proceedings. We also met for the first time a 'new' second cousin who had come to light through the internet whilst we were in Madeira. Her grandmother (Caroline) and my grandfather (Ike) were brother and sister. We spent a pleasant day with Eileen and her husband Pat at the rally and they came back to our bed and breakfast accommodation to dry out and have a look at the family tree which I had prepared.*

Monday 19th May 2003

All my coughs and colds were behind me now, I felt quite all right to travel and was invited by my friend, David and his wife, Jennifer, to accompany them to Geneva, where they were attending a trade show for the travel industry and I was taken along for the ride. Whilst there and on a gloriously sunny day, I seized the opportunity of taking a trip on one of the fine lake steamers to Yvoire in France. It was such a beautiful village, such a pity I only just had enough time to eat a crepe for lunch before heading back to the boat station. That was the last time the exhibition was held in Geneva, so unless I went as an independent traveller, I should not get to visit Yvoire again which would be a great shame, I loved it. On our last night in Geneva, we had the traditional fondue and rosti washed down with copious amounts of house red wine. I felt quite tired but knew that the following day I would be home again, so I toughed it out. There was an article in Sunday's Mail on Sunday dated 25/05/2003, it appeared that Maureen Lipman's husband Jack Rosenthal also has Multiple Myeloma, I contacted the paper and advised them of this book which in turn they said would be good to read by the Rosenthals as it gave hope to fellow sufferers, however at this juncture the book was not published so no hard copy could be sent. Jack has subsequently died of Multiple Myeloma earlier in 2004.

Saturday 7th June 2003

On what could have been my last opportunity to sail a dinghy for some time, I went down to Poole with my sailing buddy, Alan, for the usual round of sailing, beer, snooker and Chinese takeaways. We had a good sail in a fairly stiff wind and thoroughly enjoyed it, I was pleased to have done it as there may not have been another chance, every opportunity to get out and do things had to be taken.

Thursday 12th June 2003

Had to see the specialist at Worthing Hospital, my paraprotein level is up again, not a particularly good sign but I'm in no real pain so they probably will not take any action. The news is taken badly by my wife who understands the implications of this and that the cancer may be returning!

Chapter Eight.

Helping others to cope.

My wife Julie and myself were only too pleased to be able to speak to newly diagnosed Myeloma patients and their partners if invited by Dr Roques or the haematology nurse, Sarah Thompson. Some new patients want to chat and others don't because they just don't know what questions to ask or felt awkward about talking about a subject that they had previously not known anything at about, just as Julie & I did in 1998, that's why this book has been written, in response to the demand for knowledge and first hand experiences. If however the patients did finally get to meet me, most were surprised at how well I looked and that throughout the six years that I had endured the disease without too many incidents, it had rarely stopped me travelling, as the next account shows.

Friday 20th June 2003

With no secondary illness to be concerned about, we took ourselves off on holiday again and checked into the Hilton hotel at Gatwick's south terminal in readiness of flying out to Munich early the next morning. The check in at the British Airways desk was bedlam. I'd never seen so many fellow travellers at that time of morning. I was advised of a good tip that I didn't realise existed, it was to pay for the holiday by credit card and then use the 'express check in' facility at British Airways' computer terminal. It recognises the transaction and allocates seats etc. We had paid for our holiday by Switch Card rather than credit card payment, so unfortunately this facility wasn't available to us. We queued for 40 minutes and then rewarded ourselves with a cooked breakfast in the North Terminal before making our way to Passport Control. If there were more people than I expected at the check in desks, it was nothing compared to the queue for security screening! I am not a queue jumper and will be pleased to take my place in a line with the rest of my fellow passengers, however time was running out before the potential closure of our gate. Apologising profusely as we pushed our way through the milling crowds whilst trying to explain our gate was about to close, we were able to get through. How tolerant people were to a genuine need rather than some 'continental type' pushing his way forward because he'd never been brought up to queue for anything.

We made the gate by the skin of our teeth and were told that all seats had been allocated and we were having to be upgraded into business class. What a shame! The biggest shame was that we'd just paid out £15.00 for a cooked breakfast and were served another in business class, which we couldn't eat because we were full already! The flight left on time with the usual British Airways efficiency, courtesy and aplomb. We like BA for those very reasons, it's what we British do best, be good at travelling. Whilst sitting in Business Class I recognised the passenger coming through from Coach Class who wanted to use the washroom facility, it was Ron, the man we met in Madeira last Christmas who I'd known of for 30 years but he claimed not to know me. He was just as surprised to see us as we were to see him, I remarked that it seems there is no getting away from him. The flight to Munich was uneventful and some 75 minutes later we touched down and were parked up on an apron as far away from the maim terminal building as it was possible to get whilst still technically being in Germany, whilst the German flag carrier, Lufthansa enjoyed a stand at the new Terminal

2 with all the facilities within walking distance. We were allowed a few hours to ourselves before leaving to join our riverboat, so we had some time to explore Munich in the glorious June sunshine observing the Glockenspiel strike the hour and the ornate and mechanical clock at the Rathaus (Town Hall) strike another before we were driven to the pretty Austrian border town of Passau where we joined our river boat for the cruise down the Danube to Budapest. To our delight, we were joined by our 'old, new friends, Ron and Pam we had met the previous Christmas in Madeira and spent much of the cruise in their company and enjoyed the camaraderie.

We were on Viking River Cruises flagship, the *Primadonna* a recently constructed vessel built as a catamaran for stability and extra width in steel with extensive use of Formica and stainless steel for the interior, not a wooden, single hulled vessel as we were expecting, but still it was very pleasant and a thoroughly good time was had by all. One of the stops en route was the Slovakian capital of Bratislava. At a previous travel trade show attended with my friend David, I had asked a Hungarian lady what the city was like, she asked me 'Have you ever been to Crawley?' For those that have not visited Crawley in West Sussex, it became a 'new town' in the sixties and was synonymous with high rise concrete buildings of no particular architectural merit at all. This may have been 'sour grapes' as she was Hungarian and Bratislava is in Slovakia, but I was extremely surprised to find such a beautiful city where everyone was well dressed, prosperous and took pride in their city. I would gladly return and spend longer than the four hours we had there. We found that river cruising suited us very well, there are periods of inactivity whilst sailing from one docking point to the next, followed by an hour or two's sightseeing in one of the glorious and thoroughly attractive villages, many being medieval and very photogenic. Catering on riverboats is always full board and there's a risk of overeating if intake is not monitored carefully, especially when pre-breakfast coffee and Danish pastries are made available from 06:30 for the early risers and a constant stream of food was available all day long, which was devoured eagerly by some of our European cousins, but we British showed a little more decorum and ate when it was time to eat rather than just because it was there on offer.

The first 'port of call' was Melk, a very pretty village dominated by the abbey that looks out across the river. Some passengers had paid their €18 to be transported by minibus into the centre, we walked for all of ten minutes to arrive at the same time as they did. From our experience, it is seldom to any one's benefit (except the tour company) to go on an excursion if you can get there under your own steam. Half the fun of exploring new venues is to use public transport or take a taxi and go where you want to go, rather than where some one thinks you want to go. The beauty of river cruising is that you can just sit there and all the dramatic scenery comes to you, every bend opens up a new vista and all the passengers were anxious to soak up as much of it as they could. Video cameras were 'whirring', shutters clicked as life aboard ship settled into a familiar routine sailing through the night and yet another meal. We felt the need for some gentle walking exercise now to burn off some of the excess calories, but sadly the lay out of the deck doesn't allow us to 'take a turn', so we kick our heels and eagerly await our next docking which came when we arrived in the Hungarian town of Eszertagom and later at Buda-Pest. Many of the buildings on the 'Pest' side still show signs of bullet hole damage from generations of uprisings and the gentle obsolescence of neglect to this once influential Austro-Hungarian city before its unification with Buda. We made our way by taxi up to the Fisherman's Bastion which is an outstanding assortment of castellated towers and ramparts that looks out over the city of Buda to the river and Pest with its parliament building designed along the lines of London's Houses of Parliament, an impressive structure. The bastion could easily have been the underlying influence behind Walt Disney's castle in the Magic Kingdom. After dinner on board the boat, we went up to the top deck where the boat's resident organist played dance music as we sailed away into the night en route for Slovakia and Bratislava. It was one of the most memorable departures that we had ever encountered and have some excellent photographs to remind ourselves of that evening. Sometimes when I was feeling a little poorly and couldn't get out and about very far, I'd sit at my computer and watch the photographs as a slide show on my screen, or if I was in a hospital room with a television and video player I'd watch the video I recorded on our trip as it reminded me of the good times we had.

Nothing of note happened during the five days we were at home in Shoreham between our planned trips, I managed to avoid having to make a visit to the hospital. I'd stayed well and relatively pain free, I felt good and able to cope with another continental holiday so soon after coming back from the Danube cruise.

Our friends with whom we have shared many holidays don't fly so we embarked on a Wallace Arnold tour using the fast French train, the TGV down to Nice and then a short coach transfer into Italy where we stayed in Alassio. From the town we walked along the promenade to Laiguelia taking a coffee stop along the way and watched a super fit young man with a huge following of nubile young women trying to keep up with his exercise regime, it made me exhausted just to look at him. The excursion we took to Rapello and a boat trip to Portofino was the highlight of the holiday. The latter was best approached by boat as the entrance to its horse-shoe shaped harbour couldn't really be appreciated by road, which in the main by-passes the village to keep the place relatively traffic free. It had always been one of those 'must see' places and this year we achieved it. On our return to Alassio I enjoyed the last swim of the holiday followed by a soft drink and ice cream, but I was also starting to feel somewhat sore in the area of my rib cage and just hoped that it was through exercise rather than anything else more sinister.

Saturday 12th July 2003

Ribs still hurting, will be pleased to stop travelling and just get home where I can sit quietly without being jolted around. Julie's birthday today,

I'm seemingly always in trouble when there's a family birthday or wedding anniversary!

Sunday 13th July 2003

I am in absolute agony, my ribcage hurts so much the pain is indescribable. I'm being thrown about by the Michael Schumacher wannabe driver of the shuttle bus taking us back to Shoreham and I fear I've cracked some ribs as a result.

Wednesday 23th July 2003

Bad news, an x-ray at Worthing Hospital didn't reveal any cracked ribs, it was much worse. Following a week or so of taking strong pain killers and seeing the specialist, Dr Roques, he confirms that the Multiple Myelom has returned, I've relapsed. Rather disappointing as I've only been in remission for 15 months as opposed to 30 months last time. Much to consider as to best way forward from this point. I can't have another stem cell transplant and will wait to be told what drug regime will be best suited to me to arrest the cancer.

Monday 28th July 2003

Admitted to Worthing hospital and placed on a saline drip as I'm a little dehydrated. On a general ward with a promise of a cubicle when it's available.

Tuesday 29th July 2003

Starting course of steroids (Dexamethasone) and Thalidomide at just 50mg initially. Saline drip stopped as I'm suffering from sleep deprivation through having to get to pee every hour because of the excessive amount of fluid they are pumping into me. Thalidomide was used forty years ago by pregnant women as an anti-sickness drug but caused birth defects and was subsequently withdrawn from use. However, someone investigated the prospect of using it in the fight to control Multiple Myeloma as it reduces the formation of new blood vessels (angiogenesis) which Myeloma needs to grow. Because the Myeloma can't latch itself onto blood cells that don't exist, it can't grow. It does appear to work, I'm hoping that it will be as effective, particularly in my case.

Wednesday 30th July 2003

Very, very knocked out by Thalidomide, although I breakfasted, washed and dressed, I just sat in a chair, zombie like until 12:00 noon when lunch was served. It felt like being drunk but without having had the alcohol. Pain quite considerable, applied a Fentanyl patch as an alternative method of controlling the pain. May have to go to Oncology Dept in Brighton for Radiotherapy. Fentanyl was the drug used by the Russians to quell the siege at the Opera House, it killed several innocent opera goers in the process, I know how strong it is and I'm not all surprised.

Thursday 31st July 2003

Feeling very nauseous because of Fentanyl patch although pain now under control. Suffering too from some of the side effects of the Thaidomide and experiencing Tinitus.

Friday 1st August 2003

More side effects, ankles are swelling, I'm short of breath and still being sick. I'm hoping that I'll be well enough to be discharged later today as I don't have a temperature and would be better off at home. Discharged at 17:00 with lots of drugs.

Monday 4th August 2003

Pain patch removed in order to know exactly where pain is most pronounced. Due to see Dr Mitra at the Oncology Dept in Brighton at 10:10 for Radiotherapy on my ribcage.

Tuesday 12th August 2003

Dosage of Thalidomide increased to 100mg, making me feel very woolly headed and feeling quite nauseous. About to start third regime of chemotherapy, but in tablet form (Cyclophosphamide), may not suffer hair loss this time. It's not as invasive as the VAD regime and doesn't require another Hickman line being inserted into my chest.

Friday 22nd August 2003

Now that I had stopped being sick every day for the last ten days, I decided to have a last sail of the season on board the chartered yacht,

Cascade *out of Chichester Harbour. We sailed to Portsmouth Dockyard and enjoyed a lunch on board the converted* Lightship, *now painted bright green and moored in Haslar Marina close to the former submarine base. Got shooed away by the Harbour Police launch for being within 50 meters of* Ark Royal.

Wednesday 27th August 2003

Not feeling too good, being sick quite often, pain still very much in evidence, no relief yet from Radiotherapy and continuing to use pain patch as it's the strongest pain killer without going back onto Oramorph which I don't want to do. Thalidomide increased to 150 mg and making me feel very drowsy, drugged and dopey. Can't drive as too risky.

Saturday 30th August 2003

RAFA air show at Shoreham Airport, I went but didn't run around very much, just sat still and observed the aircraft, tried to drink a glass of beer but couldn't. Things must have been bad!

Wednesday 3rd September 2003

Having Pamidronate in day ward, blood tests to see if my white blood cell count is high enough for me to have more chemotherapy and will take more steroids in readiness. Paraprotein levels in urine down considerably from 10 to under 1% which is a good sign that the new regime is having some effect.

Friday 5th September 2003

Attended the Goodwood Revival meeting for vintage motor racing cars at the race track and aerodrome in Sussex. It was very noisy, and quite busy even though Friday was supposed to be the quietest day of the three day event. Spoke to Sir Stirling Moss in Lord Frederick March's private enclosure, he is a charming gentleman. I felt very tired but pleased that I'd achieved yet another excursion rather than sit at home contemplating my navel.

Monday 8th September 2003

Increased Thalidomide up to maximum of 200mg, due to be exceedingly drowsy.

Wednesday 10th September 2003

I have to attend the day ward today for a full blood count to be taken to check on my white blood cells before the chemotherapy can be administered. It's also my 59th birthday, cakes are well received by both Edburton *and* Erringham *wards.*

Thursday 11th September 2003

Having to take extra pain killers today, not feeling quite as good as I did yesterday.

Sunday 14th September 2003

Taking more steroids today in readiness for chemotherapy. I'm feeling particularly drugged today and my white cell count is probably still low because I feel feint and light headed if I bend over.

Tuesday 16th September 2003

Despite feeling a little under the weather, I attended the Southampton Boat Show as a member of the press, my sailing buddy drove us there. I didn't do too much walking about as I was still feeling a bit off, but the chance to go came up and it had to be taken.

Thursday 18th September 2003

Having to see Dr Roques in his clinic today at 12:00 noon, he'll ask for a full blood count and if it's ok I will start the chemotherapy again.

Friday 19th September 2003

I took a much promised trip on the only remaining seagoing paddle steamer, the Waverley *with my other sailing buddy. I'd been threatening to sail on her for more than 10 years and when the advert was placed in the local paper, I just had to go. We took the train from Worthing to Portsmouth Harbour which is adjacent to the berth from where the* Waverley *sails, it couldn't have been easier. It was a pleasant cruise to Yarmouth and the*

Needles off the Isle of Wight with a good hearty lunch taken on board. A good day was had by all and I was pleased to have been well enough to do it, albeit a little drowsy but as I didn't have to drive or navigate, it didn't really matter.

Tuesday 23rd September 2003

There was another helicopter trade show at Duxford, in Cambridgeshire that I was able to attend and met some of my acquaintances from Shoreham there. We stayed overnight at a Travelodge close to the aerodrome and were joined for dinner by my nephew who lived close to Stansted airport. The following day we continued up country to Norwich, revisiting the hotel in which we stayed for the wedding of our other nephew back in April and accepted the kind hospitality of the hotel for a 'free weekend' stay even though it was mid-week.

Wednesday 24th September 2003

My sister's birthday, she and her husband joined us in the evening for dinner to celebrate. We were not able to see their younger son and his wife whose wedding we attended in April, as they were flying off to Florida. We were however able to stay with our other nephew near Stansted for a couple of days on the way home to Sussex. He drove us to Cambridge and took me in a punt on the River Cam, something which I had never done before, it was quite an experience but I wouldn't have felt very safe if I had to do the punting, I'd almost certainly get the punt pole stuck in the mud or fall in and catch my death of cold, so the difficult bit was left to those who have done it before and are quite good at it.

Tuesday 30th September 2003

I feel quite rough today, I think I've got a cold coming, I hope not as it may stay with me for some time and could turn into pneumonia which would be very serious.

Thursday 2nd October 2003

I'm neutropenic, no resistance to infections as I've got no immunity system. Probably caused by low white blood cell count following my third course of Chemotherapy. My glands are up and my mouth is sore, I'm using an antiseptic mouthwash, Chlorhexidine to combat the infection which discoloured my teeth so I used smokers tooth powder to scour the stains off. I'm still feeling drugged from the Thalidomide, but not quite as bad as I have felt.

Sunday 12th October 2003

I feel really rough today, I can't turn my head quickly or bend down to tie my shoe laces in case I fall over, I feel very dizzy, drowsy and totally drugged. If I felt any worse and if it weren't for the fact that this is the weekend I'd surrender myself to the hospital. However, I'll tough it out until next week and make a decision based upon how I feel then.

Tuesday 14th October 2003

I'm due to have a bone marrow biopsy today in the day ward at Worthing Hospital. This test will determine if the cancer has been arrested. The signs are quite promising as the specialist continues to tell me how well I've responded to date from the Thalidomide, he's hopeful that all his efforts have paid dividends. I will choose to have sedation for the biopsy because it's quite painful when the auger drills into my hip bone to get at the marrow inside. Even under sedation, I have been known to swear at him, something which I would never do normally. I will not know the result for about one week.

Tuesday 21st October 2003

It's crunch day today, I'll try and intercept the specialist between his appointments to ascertain if there's any news about my biopsy. The information will be valuable as I've got to attend an appointment at Hammersmith Hospital tomorrow. Success! Dr Roques informs me that I'm in remission again. He pens a letter to Hammersmith stating that I've achieved a good 'partial' remission from the Myeloma. He can't say full remission as Myeloma may come back as to date there is no permanent cure. A copy of the letter will be sent to American Express Insurance Services to get full cover reinstated in six months time.

Wednesday 22nd October 2003

Arrived at Hammersmith to see Dr Rahmantulla, who didn't know I was coming up, what a fiasco! The upshot of it all is that we have agreed that I can take the Thalidomide for one month in three rather than constantly which would have deprived me of a quality of life, at least this way I can have two months 'to myself' inbetween courses. I feel quite good about the outcome.

I was now in remission for the third time and determined to make the most of my life. It cannot be known how long remission lasts as each time the duration in between relapses is shorter than the last time. New drugs or regimes are constantly being developed and one day a total cure will be found, until that day, we live in hope that the monthly blood tests will not reveal anything that will give rise to concern, but like the Sword of Damocles, it could have fallen at any time, without warning and caused innumerable problems again, not just for me and my family, but for the medical profession whose job it is to patch me up again and place me once more into remission. In the meantime I continued to practice what I had been preaching and travel as often as I possibly could, given that I felt well enough to do so and American Express would continue to insure me.

Help is at hand.

Currently there are over 3,600 new cases of Multiple Myeloma diagnosed annually, it is more commonly found in men than women and affects non-whites more than it does white patients, although the reason for this is not fully understood. The disease may not receive as much publicity as other blood disorders such as Leukæmia, but more and more money is being made available each year by the cancer research agencies to highlight the plight of Myeloma sufferers and to hopefully find new drugs, or to re-examine previous drugs, such as Thalidomide to combat the effect of the disease. There is still no cure currently, but one day it is hoped for a breakthrough in this area. Although a relatively new regime, Thalidomide together with Steroids and Chemotherapy, has seen a success rate of approximately 35% of patients who took part in clinical trials, being placed in remission. The sufferers of Myeloma are desperate for information, help and support. There are many cancer charities and support groups nationally offering such information, but many newly diagnosed patients often don't feel that they can come to terms with asking for information from these organisations, they would rather ask their general practitioner.

It must be said however, that many GP's hardly ever come across a case of Multiple Myeloma in their entire working life, so uncommon is the disease. It would seem unkind to say that "They wouldn't recognise a case if it hit them in the face!" but sadly it is true, they wouldn't. That is why anyone who attends their GP's clinic with a persistent back ache, must insist on being sent to the local hospital for a full blood test. It is the only way to establish if a real problem exists, without this information the doctor won't know what is the real cause of the pain or even lethargy. He can tell you to go away and rest your back, because that is what cures many of his patients, but not all. Be persistent, of course for many of you this information is too late, however it is hoped that other readers may recognise the symptoms in others and insist that they seek a thorough medical examination from someone who really knows what they are talking about. In many cases, a fellow Multiple Myeloma or Leukæmia sufferer doesn't get to know who else in their local hospital is in need of support. The nurses on the wards that deal with cancer patients, through restrictions on confidentiality, are not in a position to disclose the fact that a patient has been diagnosed with the same condition as you. Sometimes the specialists would say to the newly diagnosed patient that there is an'old hand' on the ward and would they like to talk to them. The patients, however, would appear to know amongst themselves who is a new face and who appears to be undergoing treatment, as a new 'Club Member' The obvious signs are when a Hickman line was being flushed, or of course a bald head was always a give away. Very regular checks are made on the patient's temperature, this is a sure fire way of observing if a patient has picked up an infection and is in need of a course of antibiotics to knock the temperature and the infection on the head before it becomes too severe. In many hospitals today, they use timpanic thermometers placed in the ear, as they are far more hygienic and considered more accurate than mercury thermometers. It also solves the age old problem of being given a cup of tea and then a nurse requiring a temperature reading to be taken. One elderly lady when told her temperature was to be taken was heard to say "Oh sorry dear, I've just had a cup of tea", to which the nurse quipped, "Drink it through your ear did you!", the comment fell on stony ground, or a deaf ear.

There is a very strong camaraderie between patients, almost an unwritten and unbreakable bond. It isn't restricted to patients, but also their partners, who in many cases are involved more so than the patient themselves. A recently diagnosed patient was given the opportunity of speaking with me, in a confidential manner. The Senior Hæmatology Nurse at Worthing hospital, Sarah Thompson thought it may help if the patient could get first hand information from someone who had already been through the process of chemotherapy, the side effects and the other regimes of medication. He declined the offer, either because of not wanting to ask questions which might seem to be inappropriate, or was unaware of the treatment he was about to receive and didn't want his shortcomings known, especially by a stranger. Subsequently, my wife Julie and myself were introduced to the patient's wife who by coincidence I knew from 40 years ago whilst working in Guildford. She wanted to know everything, and wasn't afraid to ask. She in turn introduced us to her husband and, from that juncture, we had maintained a high degree of contact. This I know had been more than welcomed and it had formed a friendship based upon common ground. I refer to him and others we have met as 'Cancer Club Members' and often took tea together in each others houses. Dr Roques or either of the haematology nurses often ask us, and Julie in particular, if we would 'have a word' with so and so who has just been diagnosed. We always agreed for there was no one available to talk to us from a patients point of view when I was first diagnosed. We would have welcomed it greatly, but it simply did not happen. The disease, by nature of the fact that it is as yet incurable, will not go away, neither will the dedication and support we could give each other and our partners. Dr Roques had introduced us to many couples who had just received the diagnosis, many thought that they would be 'confined to barracks' whilst undergoing treatment and were surprised to learn that I had been able to travel as extensively and that I looked comparatively well. Of courses they don't see me when I'm unwell because I was either at home 'quite lifing' or in hospital suffering from a high temperature or receiving more treatment. But all the time I can show a new patient that a positive attitude helps to get through the ordeal, I will, and hope that it does take away some of the anxieties that they may have. I had been receiving treatment for six years and had encountered most symptoms and side effects that Myeloma patients experience and as a result, Dr Roques knew there was no one better qualified to explain matters from the patient's point of view than me.

Chapter Nine.

In remission again, but for how long?

Tuesday 21st October 2003

Saw Dr Roques in his clinic and was told that I'm in remission again, albeit a partial remission.

This was obviously excellent news and gave us some encouragement, I'd been in remission on a number of occasions before and hoped that this time I could enjoy the freedom to travel that I'd previously enjoyed and advocated to other sufferers of Myeloma and other blood cancers that they should too whenever the opportunity arose. The Thalidomide dose at full strength of 200mg was knocking me about a bit, I couldn't think straight, drive, talk or as my sarcastic sailing friend said, couldn't act straight either! I was suffering from the side effects which include; tinnitus (ringing in the ears) neuropathy (trembling hands) and of course the customary constipation. Dr Roques was to ask Hammersmith if I could reduce the dose to either 100mg per day now that I was in remission, or to maintain 200mg but for one month on and two months off.

Wednesday 22nd October 2003

Having to keep an appointment at Hammersmith today with Dr Amin Rahmantulla. They still have 'overall control' of my treatment because of having two BMT's there and nothing should be done without their approval. Rather a wasted journey for although I produced the letter requesting me to attend his clinic today, neither he nor the ward clerk knew I was coming to keep an appointment. Bloods were taken and I did get to see a doctor, Dr Chan from Hong Kong who of course knew nothing about the letter that Dr Roques had sent suggesting a different dosage for my Thalidomide. So I did what I've always done when unable to get a definite answer out of anyone, I did what I thought best, which on this occasion was to keep taking Thalidomide at a constant level of 100mg to avoid the highs and lows of high dosage and then nothing for two months. Dr Roques however wanted me to carry on as prescribed until he heard something from Hammersmith or got fed up with waiting and let me do what I had proposed in the first place!

Thursday 30th October 2003

Been feeling rather light headed recently. Saw Dr Roques who checked my blood count and said that I was all right, no cause for concern.

I made a personal observation in my diary that I might have been feeling dizzy because my white blood cell count may have been low, which if so would also have the effect of impairing my already reduced immune system. However as Dr Roques did not ask for a full blood count to be conducted, it was assumed that my count was alright. But the patient knows how well his body feels and also has a fair idea of what causes problems. The hospital staff have had to take notice of my diagnosis on many occasions and know that I don't exaggerate. I'm not an armchair self diagnosis patient who reads the entire set of medical journals and imagines that I've all sorts of illnesses and conditions.

Monday 3rd November 2003

Appointment with dentist to keep mouth sweet and clean, can't afford infections of the mouth, using a strong anti-gingivitis mouth wash prescribed by the hospital. This will discolour my teeth and I'll use smoker's toothpaste to polish them up again.

Wednesday 5th November 2003

Day ward for usual Pamidronate infusion. This locks in the calcium in my bones and has helped me a great deal since taking it for over five years. Last night of 200mg Thalidomide, may start to feel more awake and 'with it' tomorrow.

Friday 7th November 2003

Not feeling quite as drugged now as the Thalidomide has been stopped since Wednesday. Not driving again yet though.

Tuesday 11th November 2003

Back and rib cage hurting again, having to take pain killers to quell it, hope it doesn't signify anything! Temperature up to 37.9, it's getting to the point when I have to notify the hospital and pack a bag.

Sunday 16th November 2003

Feeling very 'coldy' and coughing like crazy, may have to do something about it, like advise the day ward or Dr Roques.

Tuesday 18th November 2003

Surrendered myself to the system, got admitted to Erringham ward at Worthing hospital and put into cubicle 3. Temperature was 38.1, sufficiently high enough to warrant starting intravenous antibiotics. Given gentamycin and timentim, affectionately known to us chaps in the Cancer Club as our 'G and T'. Neutrophils very low at 0.06 so I'm neutropenic. (No immune system to speak of), the count should be at least 2.00

Thursday 20th November 2003

No real improvement. Will have to continue with antibiotics over the weekend in hospital. Canular broke down and needed replacing so yet another bruise to display.

Monday 24th November 2003

I'm still coughing a little but my temperature has moderated, hopefully I can be discharged today.

Wednesday 26th November 2003

Would like to say that I feel all right, but I don't, antibiotics are taking a long time to work.

Tuesday 2nd December 2003

My friend David had invited me to attend a meeting with him in Florence, I didn't accept for a number of reasons; mainly through having no immune system, it's very tiring at these shows and Italy can be quite cold in December, apart from anything else I just didn't feel up to it and felt I couldn't cope with the travelling, so I stayed home in the warm!

I'm not the only one with a cough, Julie and I sometimes walk the rescue dogs from the nearby Dogs Trust kennels, however we couldn't take any dogs out because they've got kennel cough, I wonder if that's what I had!

Monday 8th December 2003

Now that I was over the worst of the coughs and colds of the previous few weeks, we booked up to spend Christmas in Madeira again. We ordered the currency from our very helpful sub-postmaster in Shoreham and collect the Euros from him and the flight tickets from Co-op Travelcare a few days later. We couldn't wait to be back in a warm climate. We know the island quite well now as it's our third time of visiting. We flew out on Monday 22nd December, it was a rather turbulent flight and not all pilots are qualified to land at the island's extended airport at Funchal, a full Captain's licence has to be held, so dangerous is the landing strip considered to be. Some ducked out and flew on to the Canaries or Portugal, we however had a local pilot who was not in the least bit concerned that it was windy, he's used to it. A round of cheers went up on landing however and I expect a round of drinks was probably imbibed in the airport terminal bar too!

A nice week was spent in Funchal and surrounding locations with our daughter and son-in-law who was dragged up the cable car to Monte whilst our daughter soaked up the sun's rays beside the swimming pool.

As a birthday treat for our daughter we take the famous tea at Reid's Palace overlooking the harbour, at €20 a head for tea and a few cakes and finger sandwiches you would expect to have your appetite reasonably satiated, however we were all still left wanting more and thought that it was a bit of a tourist 'rip off'. Last time Julie and myself were there, we were guests of the management and the wonderfully prepared finger buffet food kept coming in abundant supply, this time it was a very different story, they didn't have to impress anyone and we were just ordinary visitors wishing to take tea at Reid's. When we returned home to England on New Year's Eve, the climate felt very different to us, it was unfamiliarly cold and on entering the house, it felt very cold too after being closed up for two weeks without any substantial degree of central heating on. We wanted to return straight away to Madeira to be in such a warm and pleasant environment, however, we would have to wait until next Spring before we would be able to travel to a warmer climate again.

New Year's Day 2004

It's a new year and lets hope that I can stay well enough to travel around a bit. I start the Thalidomide again at just 100mg and have to step up the dose in stages until I reach 200mg again, that will make me 'not quite with it' again and constantly feeling very drugged and dopey.

January 7th 2004

Appointment in the new day ward for Pamidronate to keep my calcium levels up. The department moved downstairs to be nearer to the pathology unit and the specialist who administers the treatment.

January 10th 2004

It's our son-in-law Dan's birthday and for once I was not in hospital during a family celebration, I hoped it stayed that way. However I did feel very bloated from the steroid drugs, short of breath and constipated from the Thalidomide, apart from that I was fine and I was still in remission, although at every clinic appointment and every 24 hr urine save I was expecting to be given bad news again. I even attempted to do some light interior painting, it took ages but there was no hurry, it could be done a little at a time.

In early February my friend David said he was attending a function at Olympia in London and would I like a change of scenery? I'm to go up by train, stay overnight at the Washington hotel in Mayfair and return the next day. It was a tiring two days but enjoyable none the less and I was pleased to be able to still get out and about. The friends we met on the Danube cruise had been to Tunisia over Christmas and invited their family and other friends to join them at home for a 'Tunisian Evening' They had transformed their dining-room into a Bedouin tent and made dishes you associate with North Africa. We had a great time playing games but I got very tired indeed and came away relatively early.

During the same week the flight tickets arrived from the travel agent for our trip to Florida in April, the travel insurance company had been primed up to my current situation and state of health and gave me the go ahead, we kept our fingers crossed. In readiness for hiring a car in America I thought I'd better have a new style driver's licence with my photo on it instead of the rather dog eared paper version that has seen the inside of a washing machine on more that one occasion. Using my digital camera I took a reasonable photo, printed it out and presented it, the completed application forms and myself at the relevant office in Brighton only to be told that the background colour of the photo was too pale and I'd have to have another picture taken. "There's a photo booth at the railway station round the corner" I was told, trouble was I had no cash on me so had to trudge down to the bank to use the ATM. At the bank, what bank? I hadn't been to Brighton for so long it was now a sports shop and the nearest branch of NatWest was half a mile away. What started out as a five minute job had turned into a morning's work, I was totally exhausted by the end of it and needed a sit down to recover my composure but at least I got a new driver's licence for America.

Later in February my friend David asked me to attend another travel trade show with him London and that we were to stay overnight at the Novotel in Hammersmith. This brought back vivid memories of my two bone marrow transplants at Hammersmith hospital just a couple of miles away from the hotel.

I had always had a great deal of difficulty in differentiating between the words 'hotel and hospital' and often confuse them, particularly when I was in hospital at Worthing, not only because the words sound similar but where else can you have a penthouse room with en suite facilities, sea views, room service for meals and fresh tea and coffee brought to you every two hours?

Saturday 6th March 2004

My throat is a little sore and 'tickly'. I'm coughing well and it's hurting my rib cage. Think I may have cracked a rib or two coughing, will ask Dr Roques to organise an x-ray to check it out.

I made a personal note in my diary that this could be the end of my period in remission, if so it was very disappointing because I'd only been in remission for about six months.

Sunday 7th March 2004

My ribs are hurting so much now, having to take co-codamol for pain relief in addition to dihydrocodine.

Monday 8th March 2004

Pain so severe had to ring the day ward for advice. Went into ward at noon, they took blood samples and a urine test. Had an x-ray at 16:30 but Dr Roques says no broken ribs. THIS CAN ONLY MEAN ONE THING!

Thursday 11th March 2004

Dr Roques confirms that my protein levels in the urine are up to 3.5, much higher they should be. May have to start chemotherapy again.

Wednesday 17th March 2004

Dr Roques states that the Myeloma is returning and that today I should start a new course of tablet form chemotherapy in addition to the Thalidomide. This had obviously meant that our planned trip to Florida was not a possibility for a number of reasons including not feeling well enough and travelling against the advice of my doctor which would have caused a major problem if an insurance claim had to be made whilst I was in

America. I contacted the insurance company to ask for a claim form to get the flight ticket costs refunded and phoned the travel agent to cancel the car hire arrangement. Naturally, we were devastated at having to do this but there was no other option other than to be totally sensible about the whole thing, and besides America will still be there when I'm ready to revisit.

Friday 26th March 2004

Feeling a bit off today as dosage of Thalidomide has been back up to full strength of 200mg for the last few days, not really able to walk in a straight line and slurring my words, feeling rather nauseous and have griping wind caused by the constipation through being on high dose Thalidomide.

Monday 29th March 2004

Due to start third round of chemotherapy today but have to get my blood count checked in day ward first to ensure that I'm ok to continue the treatment. All blood counts are in order so I start the chemo.

Thursday 8th April 2004

Saw Dr Roques in his clinic, he says I'm responding well to treatment, pain not as bad now that I'm receiving all the drugs. There is a strong taste of 'metal' or 'rock salt' in my mouth from the chemo, it makes me feel off and I don't want to eat, my weight is dropping.

Monday 12th April 2004

Dr Roques has put me on steroids to help boost my appetite and assist the drugs in working for me rather than against me. He asks me to conduct another 24 hour urine save to measure the protein levels. I have some pain in my hips and lower back, nothing significant but I feel slightly off because of it.

Friday 16th April 2004

Have now lost a stone in weight, I'm now down to 10.8. I've just found a lump the size of an egg in my neck at the base where it joins the shoulder blade. This could be serious! It came up very suddenly and gave me no indication at all that it was manifesting itself.

A personal observation written in my diary following this event is that this was the first real sign of the disease's progression, and it was not a good sign. Although I had come to terms with falling in and out of remission, this was something different again. I then had to wait and see what else happened to me or my condition over the next few months. It was perhaps, in hindsight a good job that this did not occur whilst we were in America, the dates would have been right and had it not been for Dr Roques saying that he didn't want me to travel so far and be unavailable for treatment for three weeks, we would have been worried sick if the lump had been found whilst so far away from the safety of Worthing hospital and the specialists there.

Sunday 18th April 2004

I feel very light headed and on the point of fainting, it may be the chemotherapy affecting me. It was our 34th wedding anniversary on this day, I felt pleased because for once I had managed to stay out of hospital for the occasion, as I had in January for our son-in-law's birthday, I'd earned some Brownie Points.

Monday 19th April 2004

Attending Dr Roques' clinic today for him to conduct a fine needle aspiration on my lump. Temperature up slightly and got a bit of a cough.

Sunday 25th April 2004

Feeling very unwell today but trying not to let it interfere too much with my activities. The taste of the chemotherapy is very strong in my mouth, I don't want to eat, I feel sick, drugged and still a little coldy, but apart from that I'm fine! I do however think that something else is 'brewing' and wonder if not just the multiple myeloma progressing but something to do with the lymph glands.

Thursday 29th April 2004

I still feel a little under the weather, attending Dr Roques' clinic but he's on holiday so seeing Dr O'Driscoll who advises me that the lump on my neck is a malignant tumour. I'll have to start another three weeks course of chemotherapy and steroids.

Wednesday 5th May 2004.

Feeling very shaky today and quite drugged from the effects of the chemotherapy, steroids and Thalidomide together. Also feeling some muscular discomfort in my back. Having to attend day ward at 15:00 hrs for a 'radioactive' drink prior to having a C. T. scan at 16:00 hrs in Worthing Hospital. The scan results are to be presented to the radiographer, Dr Mitra from the Oncology dept. in Brighton at 17:00, however the radiographer in Worthing will not release them to me, I feel like 'Piggy in the Middle' and told the specialists so.

Dr Mitra must wait for the pictures and examines me anyway. He says he can hopefully reduce my tumour by giving it a five day course of radiotherapy and will advise me when to attend his clinic in Brighton.

A fellow sufferer and myself who had both been attending Dr Roques clinic and the day ward in Worthing for the last ten years, decided to write a joint letter to the local paper, the Shoreham Herald praising the team at Worthing and the NHS in general. We thought that it was about time somebody did instead of moaning about them, it was published not just as a letter but a half page article. It earned us both a lot of Brownie Points, thanks and cuddles (and that was just from the male nurses!) I didn't realise how much the letter had been appreciated until ten days later when I really needed the hospital's care and attention.

Saturday 8th May 2004

I still feel rather dizzy and the taste of rock salt is very strong in my mouth. I have very little energy and feel thoroughly weak, no get up and go, it's gone! My weight has now dropped to ten stone, two pounds, my trousers are falling down.

Wednesday 12th May 2004

Saw Dr Roques who says no other tumours were found from the scan. Not feeling too good at present but coping all right with back pain. I feel light headed and rather sick but managing to stay 'on the right side of the line'.

Sarah Thompson the haematology nurse has asked Julie and myself to help another new patient and his wife by explaining what treatment I've had to date and how much travelling around I'd been able to undertake whilst undergoing the drug regime. This of course we were pleased to do because apart from the nurses and doctors, there wasn't anybody else who could pass on personal experiences, there was no one to talk to us in that manner, when I was first diagnosed six years ago, to have another patient's experiences passed on to us, would have been most enlightening and useful. We did meet the couple that Sarah wanted us to chat to, they were older than ourselves, but I feel our chat was in vain, there was no feedback or even a spark of interest, I believe they had already resigned themselves to the fact that, if there's no cure in sight, then there's no hope! We haven't heard from them, or even seen them in hospital again. The only 'advice' I ever received from another patient was to suck boiled minted sweets and don't let the nurses know you've smuggled in alcohol! When the nurses asked him how his fluid intake had been for the day, he told them two litres plus which met with their approval, what he didn't tell them was it was beer and gin and tonic!

Monday 17th May 2004

I feel very poorly today, constipated, nauseous, light headed and the taste of the chemo is making me be on the point of of being sick. I don't want to eat or drink and collapsed on the bathroom floor, I'm not at all well. All chemotherapy and Thalidomide is to be suspended until I recover sufficiently. Julie took me to Worthing hospital to the haematology clinic and explained to the receptionist that I needed to see a doctor very soon rather than waiting for a slot in the clinic's diary. No sooner said than done, my friend Lorraine the phlebotomist called me in straight away for blood samples to be taken and ushered me into a quite room to await the imminent arrival of a doctor.

Doctor O'Driscoll was very good, she broke off from her clinic and saw me almost immediately, she took one look at me and said 'You're staying in hospital for a few days!'

I didn't protest, I was too poorly. She phoned the bed manager who informed her that there were no beds to be had in the entire hospital. At this point Dr O'Driscoll rang Erringham ward who normally receive me to 'sort me out' on hearing that it was me who needed a bed urgently she was told to give the ward sister an hour and there'll be a cubicle available. Obviously the letter of praise to the local paper had earned me more Brownie points than I had realised! I was admitted later that day and immediately put onto a saline drip. I was still very constipated from the Thalidomide and was given Sennacot to help me, which occurred in the wee small hours of that night. I now know exactly how John Hurt felt when the alien being left his body in the film Alien.

Wednesday 19th May 2004

I've been re-hydrated, bowels sorted out and feel much better, no need to bed block, so I am discharged late in the afternoon.

Saturday 22nd May 2004

As I had remained well since my discharge I felt it was in order for us to travel up to a narrow boat festival in Rickmansworth to meet my second cousin Eileen and her husband Patrick and to meet up with the owner of my grandfather's boat Arcturus *again. The weather was much kinder to us this year, it rained non-stop at last year's festival.*

Monday 24th May 2004

I have to commence radiotherapy on my malignant tumour today in Brighton. Due to be in Dr Mitra's clinic for 16:00, the treatment was quick and we were out in half an hour but must present myself each day this week. The process is very straight forward and entails lying on the couch whilst the operator puts a lead lined patch over the area not to be blasted with radiation. They press a button and within a minute it's all over, no pain, no discomfort.

Friday 28th May 2004

Last dose of radiotherapy due today, my weight has now dropped down to 10 stones, I haven't been this weight for thirty years. I'm being prescribed different steroids following the radiotherapy and must carry a 'user's card' around with me in case I'm ever admitted to a different hospital, the steroids can't be stopped and the course must be completed at all costs, sounds very dramatic.

Another personal observation was entered into my diary;

'It has taken two weeks for the effects of the 200mg dose of Thalidomide to work it's way out of my system. I no longer feel as drugged although I expect to re-commence the drug at 100mg soon as a maintenance dose. The tablet form of chemotherapy and steroids has also stopped.'

Sunday 30th May

Jack Rosenthal died from Multiple Myeloma, I had previously written to him and his wife Maureen Lipman offering them a chance to read this book in case it gave them some encouragement, but an answer was never received.

Thursday 3rd June 2004

Seeing Dr Roques in his clinic today. Lump seems smaller now through radiotherapy, he should be pleased with my progress.

Sunday 6th June 2004

My lump is much smaller now, I'm feeling a little muzzy as I'm back on 100mg of Thalidomide. Dr Roques says I'm in partial remission. This is a major landmark and heralds the event of being able to travel again. A statement that I'm in partial remission is music to my ears, I can now perhaps re-book our flight tickets to America for September this year. It was a nautical week-end over the days of the 11th and 12th of June. I had a sail from Chichester Harbour in a ten metre yacht and a trip around Sovereign Harbour at Eastbourne on the Saturday. My motto has always been 'If you feel well enough to do it, do it for tomorrow may be too late!'.

In readiness for being able to travel abroad again, I spoke to an alternative travel insurance company as the previous two have declined to insure me once they knew the extent of the condition I'm suffering from and that I intend to travel to America, it would probably be easier to get cover to travel to the Moon than the USA, particularly as they wanted to impose a £10,000 excess on the policy, naturally I declined their offer.

However, Age Concern knew all about me, they knew the risks and were prepared to insure me and only impose an excess of £250, so all in all quite a good deal. I don't need cover however for the next planned trip up to Warwickshire to see old friends and my 'girl friend' Angela Franklin, Tony Clewett from Northampton who used to live in Richmond Road where Angela and myself lived a few doors apart, we also met up with Jean and Hilary from Northampton too, who we met on holiday in Morocco in 2001. We stayed at Wharf Cottage at Stoke Bruerne for some of the time, the owner's husband David Blagrove worked along side my grandfather Isaac Merchant many years ago at the Braunston docks, David now writes informative books about the canals of the midlands and of Braunston in particular.

Monday 14th June 2004

I was still feeling quite well and able to undertake the short break. Our daughter had arranged for us all to stay in an 'Executive Style Villa' within the Centreparc complex in Longleat Forest. It wasn't what any of us were expecting! For 'Villa' read 'Pre-Fab', for 'Executive' read 'Council House' fittings, we shall not be going back there in a hurry. Our 'Villa' was about as far away from the restaurants and on-site shop as it's possible to get and all up very steep hills on the way back, in fairness there was a land-train but for a Myeloma sufferer with a damaged spine it was most uncomfortable. Good job our stay was for only four days, although the company did post a letter through our letter-box offering the villa for a further four days at a very reasonable price, we declined their offer and couldn't get out of there fast enough! I posted a report on my travelogue web site www.travellersworld.org.uk which explains our sojourn.

Monday 21st June 2004

I was still feeling all right so did what I'd always been advocating, travel now for tomorrow may be too late, I booked for us to fly from our local airport at Shoreham to the island of Alderney just one hour away. We booked to travel with our friends, David and Jennifer, with whom I attend the travel trade shows and our 'shared' dog Ross. We used to walk him from the rescue centre before our friends adopted him, he's quite happy to come to us to stay for a short while and treats our home as his, we love him dearly. Flights were booked for 16th July 2004.

Friday 25th June 2004

We travelled up to Rugby for the weekend and to a narrow boat festival at Braunston in celebration of the butty boat Raymond *which was the last wooden hulled narrow boat to have been built. My grandfather Isaac Mercahant took me to Braunston Docks to see her (for all boats are she) being built in 1954. As soon as the present owner of the docks, now a marina, got to hear of this he introduced us to a film crew who were there featuring Raymond and Braunston Docks. We spent an exhausting day with them charging up and down the hill between the village centre, church yard and the docks. I showed them my grandmother's cottage where a photograph was taken in 1946 showing me sitting on the front door step aged two with my arms around an orange Pomeranian dog called Tony. The film crew from Carlton wanted to replicate the event and sought permission from the property owner to film me on their door step some 58 years later. Julie and I were delighted to see the cottage, I explained to the owners where everything used to be all those years ago and told them to look out on television to see me outside their cottage at sometime in the future. At the end of the day I was totally exhausted and needed to lie down to recover, we went back to our accommodation and I slept like a baby.*

On our return to Sussex I had a day out with my sailing buddy, we went on the harbour tour boat in Chichester Harbour, had lunch at the marina and then hopped across the road to the Hawk Flying Centre. Sadly not the BAE Red Arrows' Hawks but a selection of raptors. We were given bits of meat to hold in our heavily gloved fists and the twenty pound Harris Hawks would swoop low and land on our arms to take the tid-bit, it was very good and makes you realise we are not the only species on God's earth that needs feeding.

Monday 1st July 2004

Conducted urine save and delivered it to Dr Roques who confirms that my lump is cancerous, a malignant tumour and will probably have to have more Radiotherapy at Dr Mitra's clinic in Brighton. I feel alright apart from a bit shaky from the Thalidomide.

Friday 9th July 2004

As I felt alright that day I accompanied a friend when he went to visit a work colleague in Horsham, just half an hour away by car. We chatted about life and things in general and enjoyed a lunch at a trendy wine bar, we were the oldest two guys in there so we tried not to show our selves up by ordering a Mackeson or pint of Brown and Mild, we drank Becks beer out of the bottles, I think we got away with it.

Saturday 10th July 2004

Today was the Ardingly Vintage Vehicle Show held at the renowned County Show Ground near Haywards Heath in Sussex. There were many cars of the vintage of my father's car described in chapter one. I did quite a lot of 'running around' and became quite tired, but a good night's sleep soon sorted me out again.

Sunday 11th July 2004

Despite all the activity over the last few days, I attended a local event at Shoreham Port Authority. It was an open day with RNLI lifeboats, the mine-sweeper HMS Atherton *and several other large craft and war time Motor Torpedo Boats. One of the main reasons for attending was that a nurse from the day ward in Worthing that I know so well was competing in the Dragon Boat race within the harbour and I wanted to show my support, sadly I didn't see her as all girls look the same in wet suits!*

Monday 12th July 2004

Sarah Thompson the haematology nurse rang to say that Dr Roques wants to see me, sounds a little ominous!

Thursday 15th July 2004

Saw Dr Roques in his clinic in Worthing, I'm relapsing again after just one month, I'm devastated. I knew that, as the disease progressed the periods in between remission would get shorter but I would have hoped for more than four weeks! He wants to conduct a bone marrow biopsy which entails the auger into hip again, I choose to be sedated for the operation. He also wants me to be admitted in order that full biopsy on my lump can be taken rather than the fine needle aspirations that he has conducted on two previous occasions. I will also have to be admitted on a subsequent occasion to have another Hickman line inserted, this will be my fifth in readiness to receive a new chemotherapy regime called ESHAP

Friday 16th July 2004

If I could stand up and walk unaided then I was well enough to travel! We flew with our friends and our 'shared dog' Ross from Shoreham airport to the island of Alderney in a Britten Norman Trilander aircraft, a noisy three-propelled airplane that hauled it self into the Sussex sky for the one hour flight to Alderney. I enjoyed every minute of it but those who didn't like flying were very apprehensive about it being such a small aircraft that wasn't jet propelled. We stayed in the 'capital' of the island, St Anne's which has one main street and diddley squat else. Fortunately the weather was kind to us which helped as we weren't allowed in many places with the dog who was so well behaved, he was such a good dog and didn't mind the flight at all. On the following day we took the one hour open top bus tour of the island, the driver had to stop for forty minutes at a viewing point otherwise we would have been back within twenty minutes having seen everything the island had to offer. We came straight off the bus and boarded the little train which ran for two miles up to a stone quarry. Alderney purports to be the only one of the Channel Islands which boasts a rail service, if that's what you call it. We flew home the next day having run out of things to see and do, I'm pleased we went but have no need to revisit in the immediate future.

Monday 19th July 2004

Dr Roques rang me to confirm an appoint has been made for me to attend the clinic of the Ear, Nose and Throat specialist, Mr Harries. It is he who will conduct a full biopsy on my lump when I'm admitted to Worthing hospital for the lumpectomy.

Wednesday 21st July 2004

Knowing that I was shortly to be admitted to hospital for surgery, I took the last opportunity this week to get out and about, which by now you will have realised is my advice to anyone in the same situation if they feel well enough. With my wife Julie we attended the Farnborough Air Display having driven up the night before and stayed in a Bed and Breakfast establishment that we've used on previous occasions. The show was busy and noisy and I enjoyed every minute of it, it may be the last time I can attend.

Saturday 24th July 2004

Another busy day, my sailing buddy Alan was given a flying lesson as a birthday present and today he took to the skies over Shoreham accompanied by his wife's uncle who is in his eighties and never flown and daughter-in-law who operated the video camera to record the occasion. We attended to see how they all got on and left them to it to attend our friend David's birthday party close by. We saw the dog, Ross and left when all the Pimm's punch had been drunk.

Tuesday 27th July 2004

Admitted to hospital in Worthing at 07:30 in readiness for my lumpectomy. I went to the operating theatre at 09:30 and was there until 11:00. I awoke feeling drugged and sore but otherwise alright. It'll be some time before the results are known.

Saturday 31st July 2004

I've made another personal observation in my diary that a slight niggle of pain has developed in my lower back and pelvis which can be eased at night through taking two dissoluble co-codamol tablets.

Monday 2nd August 2004

Having to attend the dentist today to ensure that there is no decay or sharp edges in my mouth which could be affected by the imminent chemotherapy.

Tuesday 3rd August 2004

I awoke with a 'squitty' tummy and my temperature is fluctuating wildly, I'm obviously attempting to fight off some bug or other. Also having to attend the local GP's surgery to enable the practice nurse to remove the stitches in my neck following the lumpectomy.

Wednesday 4th August 2004

Dr Roques has had a good look at the tissue from my lump and now proclaims it to be Non-Hodgkins Lymphoma. We are given an information booklet which confirms that it is a cancer of the lymph gland and swells because the body is fighting against it and causes enlarged lymph nodes.

As if I hadn't got enough on my plate to be concerned over, I now had a second form of cancer to monitor and worry about. The lymphoma also attacks the bone marrow and causes damage which reduces the bodies ability to produce bloods cells in sufficient numbers to fight off infections. The specialists said that chemotherapy and radiotherapy could help in getting rid of lymphoma. I had both at various intervals and could no longer receive more radiotherapy in case damage was caused to healthy tissue. Where on earth do we go from here?

Chapter Ten.

Talk of a third Bone Marrow Transplant.

Dr Roques had on more than one occasion mentioned that non Hodgkins Lymphoma could also be cured by a stem cell transplant, better known perhaps as a bone marrow transplant. He advised me that Hammersmith hospital still had some of my stem cells frozen from the original harvest conducted in 1998. He would contact the team up there and discuss the merits of me undergoing a third transplant. It should also be mentioned at this juncture that it is not common practice at all to conduct a third transplant, I felt that he only made the suggestion because I had previously responded well to any treatment administered.

Thursday 5th August 2004

Sister Cathy North rang us to say that I was to be admitted to Worthing hospital on Sunday evening, the 15th August for the insertion of a Hickman line in order to receive chemotherapy on my lump and underlying condition. This date had been previously agreed as the first available date following our very imminent holiday cruising down the Rhine, a style of holiday that we had found suits us very well as it's sedate and restful interspersed with frenetic activity for an hour or two when the boat moors up somewhere. I had been feeling quite well prior to our departure and was allowed to take the holiday with the blessing of Dr Roques, he like most other people connected with my treatment knew that I would never travel anywhere if it wasn't approved of. I am pleased to record that permission was granted and in accordance with my own dictate of travelling whilst I felt up to it, we went.

So imminent was it that later that same day the taxi arrived to take us to the railway station for the train up to Gatwick airport. We weren't actually flying out until the next morning but we don't like rushing about at 'cock crow' and invariably choose to stay overnight in an airport hotel. On this occasion it was le Meridien at the airport's North Terminal.

Friday 6th August 2004

Fortunately BA had allowed us to check our baggage in the night before as ours was the first flight out to Amsterdam the next day. All we had to do was saunter through Passport Control and watch the indicator boards for a boarding gate number. We took off at 07:30 and arrived at Amsterdam's Schiphol airport at 09:30 local time and in glorious sunshine. We were met by a DMC (Destination Management Consultant) and put onto the shuttle bus which served four or five hotels in the area of the airport. We stayed at the Ibis, a three star hotel of enormous proportions, but no air conditioning to speak of, which was a shame because it really was hot at 30 degrees.

We had never been to Amsterdam before so it was an ideal opportunity to do some sightseeing before we picked up the coach to take us to the boat the next day. We retraced our steps on the shuttle bus which took us back to the airport from where there was a fast and frequent rail service into the city centre. We buddied up with an American couple who were on a punishing tour of Europe, 'If it's Friday this must be Amsterdam!' We journeyed together as four sets of eyes are better than two when attempting not to get too lost. It didn't work, we still got lost because we got on the wrong train. They had pre-booked a two hour coach tour of the city and tagged along because it would have been too hot to walk around aimlessly. We shall never meet again but our day was made through being in their company, that is what travel is all about, meeting people and getting to know them briefly before saying our good byes.

Saturday 7th August 2004

I took only a low dose of 50mg of Thalidomide as I didn't want to be too drowsy for the duration of the holiday. Boats have gang-planks and I didn't want to play Capt. Hook falling into the water.

The coach company collected us from the Ibis and drove to Arnhem to pick up the boat, there was no time for sight seeing, the Princess Christina was waiting for us and the other 100 passengers made up of us Brits and the Dutch who turned out to be just as noisy and assertive as the Germans had been on our river cruise last year. But we co-existed with them well enough for the week we were together although it was very peaceful when we had the boat to ourselves for one night at the end of the cruise. We even met again a couple who were on the Danube trip last year, we recognised each other immediately, it's such a small world.

The first town we moored up at was Homberg where the hats were made, or at least were named after. Famous wearers of such headgear were Neville Chamberlain and Tony Hancock. There was absolutely nothing to capture our imagination in this sleepy town, we walked by the river after dinner and saw no one except our fellow passengers. A large cast iron plaque on the wall showed the levels to which the Rhine had risen in previous years, perhaps all the town's inhabitants had been washed out of their houses, never to return.

Sunday 8th August 2004

The lymphoma lump on my neck feels very sore this morning, I decide to dissolve two co-codamol tablets to ease the pain, I may have to take more at bedtime tonight. The boat sailed onto Cologne during the morning, this stretch of the Rhine is not pretty at all and quite boring unless you like petrochemical refineries and gravel silos. The tour company should have flown us to Cologne airport and commenced the cruise from there, this is a waste of two days sailing. The cathedral at Cologne is very impressive and right in the centre of the city, most other streets leading away from it were full of the usual high street names and not quaint streets to capture the travellers imagination, we left it with no intention of returning.

Monday 9th August 2004

Pain in neck region still quite uncomfortable so took more co-codamol. I don't feel poorly, just aware of this enlarged lymph gland.

The boat left its dock at 05:00 en route to Andernach, which was an interesting town with a walled fortification, interesting streets and wonderful cake shops. It was also very hot there and drained my strength, I claimed that I was 'Andernachered' by the end of the day. It was the captain's birthday and in the evening the crew threw a barbecue for him, the passengers were not invited but we might just as well have been there as it was held on the grass bank immediately adjacent to the boat and we caught all the cooking smells and the popping of corks.

Tuesday 10th August 2004

My lump is hurting even more now, it prickles and stings. I will be glad to be admitted to hospital upon my return so that the chemotherapy treatment can commence. What a statement to have made, being glad to go into hospital! I didn't feel unwell with my lymphoma, just very uncomfortable and know that was the 'safest' place to be, under the care and supervision of the team at Worthing hospital. In the meantime we had a holiday to enjoy, the cruise boat arrived in Rudesheim at lunchtime. For those who have not yet visited this delightful German town, it's a medieval town with wonderful half timbered buildings, most of which are in Drosselgasse Street. There are bars and restaurants which attract visitors as though there's no tomorrow. Our boat was moored quite close to the main part of town so we bought cakes from the local baker and returned to our cabin, made tea and had a well deserved rest. Later that day we saw our first spot of rain which prevented us from exploring again after dinner, not that we needed much encouragement to stay on the vessel, it was very comfortable.

Wednesday 11th August 2004

I've developed a silly tickle in my throat, I'm putting it down to the enlarged lymph gland pressing on the throat which has never been the same since my first bone marrow transplant when my throat closed completely due to the mucusitis. The boat had turned around at this point and we were on the return leg of the journey. We moored at Koblenz which is at the confluence of the Rhine and Mosel rivers, the latter being much more attractive than the former. We attempted to join an organised coach tour from Koblenz to Cochem which also is considered to be an attractive town to spend some time, but we shall never know as we couldn't get there. Unfortunately all seats were taken and there were insufficient numbers of additional passengers to justify the expense of hiring a mini-coach, so we missed out on that trip which was a great shame. I was feeling good and could have coped with the coach journey and cable car ride over the vineyards up to the viewing point high above the Mosel river, I'll have to put it on my list of things to do next time.

Thursday 12th August 2004

I still feel all right except for my lump, it stings and necessitates taking two co-codamol four times a day just to ease the discomfort. The boat had moored up at Dusseldorf in the pouring rain so we waited until the sun shone before venturing out to explore the city, we didn't have to wait long. It's a vibrant place, nicer than Cologne as it had a homely atmosphere and designer boutique shops rather than the chain stores that we encountered in Cologne.

Friday 13th August 2004

I am not a superstitious person by nature, so the date doesn't have a real significance. I will however be pleased when tomorrow comes because it'll mean we're flying home. My tickly throat still catches me out during conversations but apart from that I still feel alright with the exception of a few sneezes every now and then.

The boat had arrived back in Arnhem and we said our good byes to the Dutch passengers that we had come to know during the past week, they were a pleasant group once you got to know them. The boat seemed very quiet that evening after their departure. Disembarkation took quite a while and was mainly in the rain but it didn't stop some of our more robust passengers being dockside to see them depart and to take a short walk along the riverside, we stayed on board in the dry. We retired to bed early that night as we were disembarking early the next day ourselves en route to the airport at Amsterdam.

Saturday 14th August 2004

I've survived a ten day holiday without mishap and feel safe now in the knowledge that England is only an hour's flight away.

It seemed a pity to have wished our time away by counting the hours before I would be admitted to hospital, it's a difficult concept to follow for those who have never been in the position of vulnerability health wise. Also my mind went back to the time that I was feeling unwell in Italy and had to be flown home, it's much better to think that you survived for a time on your own without having to rely upon others to get you out of trouble.

The tour coach arrived at the boat at 08:00 to drive us to Schiphol Airport for our flight home at 12:45 local time, we touched down at London Gatwick at 12:20 and we were home in Shoreham by 15:00, all safe and sound.

Whilst away I made a personal observation in my diary that the crick in my neck that I reported to Dr Roques in June may very well have been the start of the lymph gland swelling and that the silly tickle in my throat may well have been the start of a chest infection that would ultimately see me in hospital for longer than I had imagined.

Sunday 15th August 2004

This was the last day of the Eastbourne Air Show which I didn't want to miss as I knew that the following day would see me in hospital for a week or ten days. We only stayed at the show for two or three hours, I began to feel unwell and so returned home as soon as possible.

I have started to shake and shiver which can only mean one thing, I've got a chest infection. On reaching home I check my temperature which is 38.9 degrees and has to be reported to the hospital. I receive the answer I was expecting, 'Pack a bag Peter, you're coming in!' On arrival at hospital I was given dissoluble Paracetamol to reduce the temperature, clerked in and given a bed. A nursing sister installed a canular and administered Augmentin as an antibiotic to reduce the effects of the infection.

Monday 16th August 2004

In readiness to receive my Hickman line in an operation later today, I was asked to have a medication based shower to ensure that there was no skin flora on me, I await instructions. The specialist advised me that he wouldn't advise the insertion of the new line today as it would be pointless in doing so if I had a chest infection, better to wait until it had cleared up, I agreed wholeheartedly as I didn't want the new line being infected as soon as it was installed. I was also asked to remove myself from cubicle 4 and go back into a general ward as someone more poorly than myself needed it. I did so willingly as it's what I would expect others to do for me if I needed the safety of a cubicle, especially if I was neutropenic (no immune system).

A sad day as one of the other 'Cancer Club' patients died, it was his wife, Flick, who I knew in Guildford 40 years ago who told us, I couldn't attend Tony's funeral as I was an in-patient, Flick knew this and appreciated the situation.

Tuesday 17th August 2004

I'm feeling a little poorly today, my temperature is still up and my lump on the neck is hurting so I took two co-codamol to ease the pain and hopefully reduce the temperature, although Paracetamol is normally prescribed. My temperature at noon is 38.4 degrees, far too high for comfort and may well be caused by an infection which occurred when they put in the canula, I'm told it's a staphylococcus flora of the skin. Therefore it'll delay the operation and receiving of chemotherapy until the bug is cleared up through the use of antibiotics. I am hoping to get home by Thursday with tablet form of antibiotics and return next week for the operation, we'll have to see.

Wednesday 18th August 2004

I feel quite good on waking, the co-codamol helped me rest more easily in my bed. Also because I haven't been taking Thalidomide since last Sunday, I don't feel drugged. At 06:00 I was given my first intravenous antibiotic (Cefuroxine) of the day to clear up the chest infection. My temperature is coming down now but I still have to keep it within acceptable parameters before the Hickman line can be inserted.

Thursday 19th August 2004

My lump feels so large now and it hurts, I'm having to take co-codamol every four hours now to get some relief from the pain. A full blood culture sample was taken this morning to see how my two infections are doing and as I'm being prescribed Gentamycin and Timentin, known to us patients as 'G and T', I assume that the infections are still very much in evidence. My temperature is still not under control and I had a 'spike' when it rose again to 38.3 and on subsiding it caused me to have the rigours. I ask for Pethadine to quell the shaking, it's the only thing that really works. I am not a happy bunny! As you might expect, I didn't go home.

Friday 20th August 2004

The pain is no less, in fact it's getting worse. I haven't felt this uncomfortable for about four years and having to increase my Dihydrocodine and ask for Oramorph (liquid morphine).

Saturday 21st August 2004

Some advice given to me now from a senior nurse, 'why not ask the doctor to put you on steroids again, it might just work!'. The doctor agreed and I start a course of Pregnoselone in the hopes that it does help, it certainly won't do any harm.

Sunday 22nd August 2004

Another canula had to be inserted in my hand as the previous one collapsed, more skin punctures and bruising. My skin feels very itchy today although my temperature seems to be subsiding a little. I decide to call my lump Zaphod Beeblebrox after the character who had a second head in Douglas Adams' classic book the Hitchhiker's Guide to the Galaxy.

Monday 23rd August 2004

I've seen all the doctors in the team looking after me and I can have the operation to insert the Hickman line tomorrow which means Nil by mouth from midnight tonight.

Tuesday 24th August 2004

I am being allowed the smallest sips of water before being taken down to the operating theatre, as yet I don't know at what time it'll be, but I put on the back to front hospital gown in readiness. I'm collected at 11:00 and wheeled into the pre-op room and immediately see the friend who we cruised down the Danube last year, we keep meeting in all sorts of odd places as neither of us knew that the other would be in hospital. I'm back in my bed on the general ward at 13:00 and feel rather sore where the line went in. At least I'm now balanced as far as pain goes as I've got the lump on my left side of my neck where it meets the chest and the Hickman line on the right side of my chest. I missed lunch, thank goodness! I have to start a serious programme of hydration to ensure that no damage is caused to my kidneys when I commence the chemotherapy treatment tomorrow.

Wednesday 25th August 2004

The day has come when my chemotherapy treatment can commence.

I am to receive a regime called ESHAP or indeed a modified form of it.

On day one, I am to receive:

40mg of etoposide, which is chemotherapy, over one hour through my line.

500mg of the steroid methyl-prednisolone over 30 minutes.

2mg in 500mls of the chemotherapy, cytarabine over three hours and 25 mg in 1000mls of saline of the chemotherapy cisplatin over 24 hours which has to be delivered through just one of the three lumens on my Hickman line, no others can be used. Hydration has to continue throughout the treatment.

Thursday 26th August 2004

I am to receive all of the above mentioned drugs in the ESHAP regime with the exception of cytarabine which was a one dose only drug. This treatment was conducted in the day ward because it's very labour intensive and needs the continuity of nursing attention. I was transferred into cubicle 3 on Erringham ward on the fourth floor and had to keep reminding everyone that the toilet didn't work. After 24 hours I gave them an ultimatum, get it fixed or I call in a plumber myself, it was fixed in half an hour.

Friday 27th August 2004

Another all day visit to the day ward for ESHAP and a blood transfusion to perk me up a little as I am beginning to feel a little off through the effects of the chemotherapy. Tomorrow I must remain in my cubicle for the chemo as the day ward is not open at weekends, I'll lose continuity of attention.

Saturday 28th August 2004

Just as I predicted, no co-ordination when chemo is to be administered. The regular nursing staff are not qualified to give ESHAP, it has to be given by a Clinical Nursing Sister. Unfortunately I do not have sole possession of this person who is in constant demand elsewhere. The etoposide element of the chemotherapy was put up on a drip stand and the promise made that within an hour it will have gone through my line. It took considerably longer than that despite my constant request that the flow rate be increased, it took five hours. This would never have happened in the day ward! I'm getting frustrated now by the lack of attention to detail and organisation, I'm an 'old hand' at managing my own illness and know what is right and what is not, this is not good practice.

Sunday 29th August 2004

I've now been in hospital for two weeks, I shall be glad to leave and believe the nursing staff that I have had to cajole into doing things properly will be pleased to see me go home too! The last of the ESHAP chemotherapy regime finished today at midnight, way, way overdue but as explained, it's the weekend and the day ward is closed. What is also exacerbating the situation is that it's a Bank Holiday, so normal services will not be resumed until Tuesday.

Monday 30th August 2004

Dr Roques rang Erringham ward to ascertain if all my bags of fluids had gone through and that I was no longer connected to a pump on a drip stand. On hearing that I was disconnected, I was given permission to go home, music to my ears. My departure was a comparatively swift procedure with envelopes of temporary support drugs given until I am able to collect my prescription from the pharmacy department on Tuesday. Normally a letter is produced and should be given to my GP, but I left in such haste that it wasn't ever produced. It wouldn't have made any difference anyway as I am never visited by the GP on discharge from hospital, he has probably lost count of the number of times I've been in and out of hospital.

Tuesday 31st August 2004

I stopped taking the Thalidomide whilst in hospital and feel quite with it at the present time, also I'm not suffering too much from the effects of the chemotherapy. My stomach is really playing up today, I fear I may be dehydrating and will have to go back in for 24 hrs whilst they re-hydrate me.

Wednesday 1st September 2004

I didn't have to go back in as an in-patient, but I do have to attend the day ward every day this week for blood samples to be taken to ensure all is well. The stitches at the entry site of Hickman are to be removed today. I have to phone in every day for this next week too to get the results of the blood tests. I have avoided being admitted for hydration and I understand my blood statistics show a daily improvement, therefore by the end of the week I'll no longer be neutropenic and will have some natural immunity back.

Thursday 9th September 2004

Today is the last day that I have to inject myself with GCFS (Granulite Stimulation Factor) to boost the growth of my white blood cells. My hair has started to fall out but I don't feel too bad from the effects of the chemotherapy, but there's time yet. My lump still hurts like crazy.

Friday 10th September 2004

Today was a very significant day in my life, it was my 60th birthday and a full day's celebrations were planned. The day started off in the usual manner at present, which entailed a visit to the day ward. We took a quantity of cakes in for the nurses and received their everlasting gratitude. A photograph was taken by my wife Julie in the day ward at Worthing

Hospital showing me and eight of the nurses immediately prior to them getting sugar on their mouths from the doughnuts we took in for them.

Saturday 11th September 2004

My lump feels bigger today and it hurts or rather stings unmercifully, I'm having to take more pain killers now to control the discomfort. I had another busy day seeing friends who were not able to join in my celebration yesterday. I retired to bed rather later than anticipated but probably slept all the better for it.

Sunday 12th September 2004

I spiked a temperature of 37.9 degrees which is only marginally short of the crucial temperature level that the hospital say I should report to them in case any thing is brewing. I took two dispersible paracetamol instead and hope that it lowers the temperature sufficiently.

Wednesday 15th September 2004

I have an appointment to attend the day ward for the removal of the stitches holding the Hickman line in place. Dr Roques observes my lump and is totally dismayed by its size and that the ESHAP chemotherapy treatment did no good at all. The line is removed as it has served its purpose and is not required again as no further treatment will be administered. I am prescribed a two week course of steroids in the hopes that it'll do some good and told to present myself to Dr Roques for him to see it on the 27th.

Today was not a good day for either my wife Julie or me, we are told that it was thought that no further treatment was available to me as I had everything and must now await someone coming up with a new regime or resurrecting an old drug, like Thalidomide which sadly did not work for me. My body would not be able to withstand the third stem cell transplant which was suggested earlier and I'd had all the radiotherapy that they could safely beam at my body without killing vital structural organs. I've had five courses of chemotherapy and survived them, I'd be pushing my luck somewhat if I underwent another bout during the stem cell transplant. I then had to resign myself to the fact that they could do nothing whatsoever in the future to help me through my cancer treatment and I had to monitor my condition best way

I could. I had suggested that as the lump had now grown to significant proportions and was clearly still visibly growing, that the radiologist should find sufficient new cancer cells to aim radiotherapy beams at without encroaching into structural tissue. It was therefore agreed that the haematology nurse at Worthing who had worked so tirelessly upon my behalf, would make this suggestion to the radiologist, Dr Mitra from Brighton who was to visit Worthing Hospital the next day.

Sarah Thompson, as good as her word did ask him and it was further agreed that he would be prepared to look at the situation in the hopes that he could find an area for the radiotherapy to be aimed at. He examined the lump and stated that he would need to check his notes in Brighton to ensure that there was still some leeway, although I could have to wait for four weeks before any treatment could be conducted because of the excessive demand upon the three radiotherapy machines.

Monday 20th September 2004

I believe that my lump has enlarged and is now pressing against my neck glands making talking a little awkward and I feel it creeping around the back of my neck. I am taking pain killers and resort at night to a low dose of Oramorph to help me through the night.

Tuesday 21st September 2004

My lump is getting larger every day now, It's quite concerning, where will it end? Phone calls from both the St Barnabas hospice nurse and the haemaotology nurse in Worthing who both think that if the control of pain is eased by the use of Morphine, then I should not stick out and be brave, but to get the relief that the opiate provides.

Wednesday 22nd September 2004

Encountered terrible pain in the right femur last night, almost certainly bone pain caused by the progression of the Myeloma, took Oramorph, little or no relief.

Thursday 23rd September 2004

I was pleasantly surprised to have received a telephone call from Dr Mitra's office in Brighton confirming that my suggestion of further treatment was a possibility and that more radiotherapy could be conducted shortly without having to wait the four weeks initially suggested. This is a significant result and offered hope once more to what was earlier a rather 'final' situation as far as further treatment was concerned. I was to attend his clinic in Brighton on the following Monday for the simulation exercise which entailed taking precise measurements of the area that is to be bombarded.

The St Barnabas Hospice nurse, Patricia makes a house call today to introduce herself and give advice on my pain control. A very informative meeting.

Friday 24th September 2004

Very, very bad pain in right femur over night, had to get out of bed and sit in a chair downstairs (will buy high back chair for bedroom tomorrow to avoid disturbing Julie whilst I avoid the creaky stairs down to the lounge. It never rains but pours, Julie's 87 year old father fell over at a tea dance and had broken his shoulder and hip bone, she was now having to be concerned over the pair of us, not just me.

Saturday 25th September 2004

Having severe problems today with double vision, images are as much as eight feet apart, not good news and needs looking at. It may be caused by the lump pressing against a nerve, can't do anything about it as it's the week-end, will have to see Dr Roques on Monday.

Monday 27th September 2004

Couldn't see Dr Roques as I'm due in Brighton to see Dr Mitra for radiotherapy at 09:00. Mentioned it to him who conducted stringent eye examination. Whilst in Brighton I had an x-ray on my right femur to ascertain the cause of the bone pain, it is revealed the there is an anomaly that will subsequently be treated with radiotherapy, but not now, at a later date, but soonish. Dr Mitra also suggested that an MRI brain scan be conducted at some time in the near future to check for brain tumours causing the double vision.

Tuesday 28th September 2004

Commenced first round of radiotherapy on neck lump at 12:30, more to follow during the week. Spoke to Dr Roques who had approached the Royal Marsden Hospital in London to ascertain if the alternative drug to Thalidomide, could be beneficial to me. The general level of consensus is that it would not help me and cause 'more trouble than it's worth'. It does also cost £31,500 per month to prescribe!

Wednesday 29th September 2004

Today was Dr Roques' 65th birthday and I wanted to mark the occasion by presenting him with a card and present to thank him for all his kind attention and professionalism over the last six years that he had been looking after me.

He also retired on this day, but will return as a consultant, he would never have been able to just walk away from his patients after a period of 23 years, it would have been too alien to him. Later that day I also had to attend the radiotherapy clinic in Brighton for a further bout of treatment and was advised that initially that the lump will grow even larger before any appreciable difference is observed. I sincerely hope that the lump will reduce as it's sore and the scar tissue is being stretched to breaking point, sometimes it will ooze a little blood whilst I towel myself off after showering.

Thursday 30th September 2004.

Attending Brighton radiotherapy clinic for the last of this week's treatment, just Monday next week to go and a follow up 'inspection' by a doctor to see how I am coping with the radiotherapy and its side effects, which to date have been minimal, or better than that, non-existent. I also attended an appointment in Worthing with the eye specialist, Mr Clifford-Jones who after a thorough examination organised an MRI scan on my brain for next week.

Author's Note.

I sincerely hope that the book has been informative, but not so medically biased as to need a degree in medicine to read and follow my account of life at the sharp end of a needle so to speak. As previously mentioned, the book was undertaken in response to requests from doctors and specialists for a personal view on how a patient copes with a blood cancer, whether it be Multiple Myeloma, Leukaemia, Hodgkins Lymphoma or an even more rare condition, Plasma Cytoma which develops into Multiple Myeloma at some stage in the future. Newly diagnosed patients of these blood diseases sometimes hold back when asking questions of a doctor as they may not wish to show their lack of knowledge in the subject, or are just too frightened to ask. Hopefully this book will answer their questions and should be read by every person whose lives these diseases have touched, that includes their partners, children, other relatives, carers and close friends. The specialists can advise the patient what medication and procedures they will receive during their intensive period of treatment but as they haven't been through the process themselves, they can't advise the patient how they are likely to feel, I have been through the hoop and know how the new patient will feel, that's why my book should be read in the first instance after a blood cancer has been diagnosed.

End of narrative.

Useful contact names and addresses of relevant organisations

Cancerbacup
3 Bath Place
Rivington Street
London
EC2A 5JR

Telephone:	Freephone 0800 18 11 99
Website:	www.cancerbacup.org.uk

Leukaemia Care Society
14 Kingfisher Court
Venny Bridge
Pinhoe
Exeter
Devon
EX4 8JN

Telephone:	01392 464848

Hodgkin's Disease Association
PO Box 275
Haddenham
Aylesbury
Bucks.
HP17 8JJ
Telephone: 01844 291500

Cancerlink
11-21 Northdown Street
London
N1 9BN Telephone: 0207 833 2818
Facsimile: 0207 833 4963
Email: cancerlink@canlink.demon.co.uk

Editor's Note

My dear friend Peter Berry, passed away on the Fourth of October 2004. Throughout his terrible illness, Peter never for a moment lost his brilliant sense of humour, always having something very witty to say when we spoke on the phone or communicated by e-mail. He is missed by everyone whose life he touched.

David Aherne.

Finally

Some of Peter's travel features can be found on www.global-traveller.net including "Ashes to Lemons".

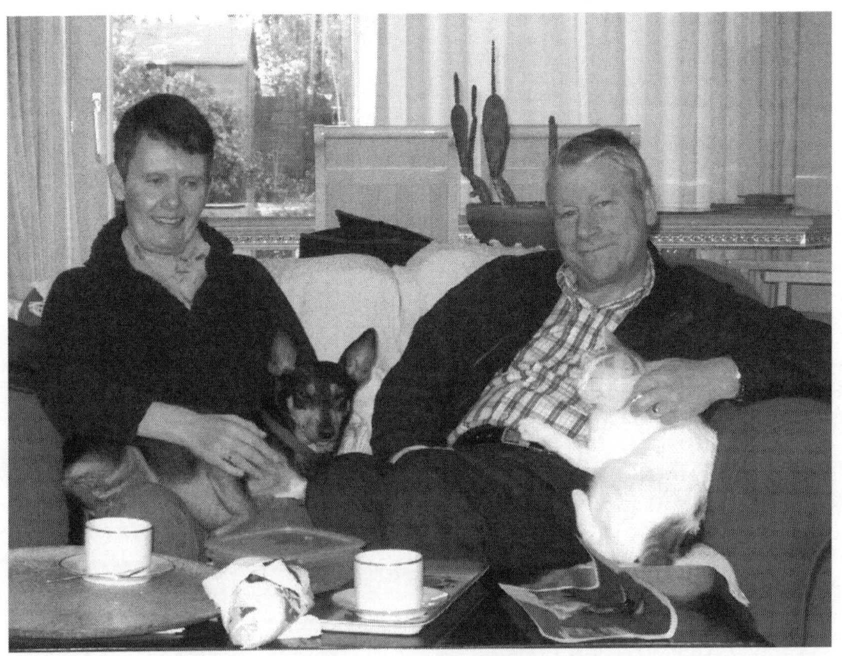

Julie, Peter, Ross and Fruitcake the cat